Complete Con
ICE HOCKEY

Complete Conditioning for
ICE HOCKEY

Peter Twist, MPE
Strength and Conditioning Coach
Vancouver Canucks

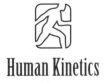

Human Kinetics

Library of Congress Cataloging-in-Publication Data

Twist, Peter, 1963-
   Complete conditioning for ice hockey / Peter Twist.
     p.   cm.
   ISBN 0-87322-887-1
   1. Hockey--Training.   2. Physical fitness.   I. Title.
   GV848.3.T85   1996
   796.962'07--dc20

                                      96-8062
                                       CIP

ISBN: 0-87322-887-1

Photo on page 2 courtesy of Carlos Amat. Photos on pages 10 and 22 courtesy of Vancouver Canucks/Kent Kallberg. Photo on page 67 courtesy of Toronto Maple Leafs/Graig Abel. All other interior photos courtesy of Vancouver Canucks/Jack Murray.

Developmental Editor: Kirby Mittelmeier; **Assistant Editor:** Chad Johnson; **Editorial Assistant:** Amy Carnes; **Copyeditor:** John Wentworth; **Proofreader:** Bob Replinger; **Graphic Artist:** Angela K. Snyder; **Graphic Designer:** Stuart Cartwright; **Photo Editor:** Boyd La Foon; **Cover Designer:** Jack Davis; **Photographer (cover):** Courtesy of Vancouver Canucks and Orca Bay Sports & Entertainment/Jeff Vinnick; **Illustrator:** Studio 2-D; **Printer:** United Graphics

Human Kinetics books are available at special discounts for bulk purchase. Special editions or book excerpts can also be created to specification. For details, contact the Special Sales Manager at Human Kinetics.

Printed in the United States of America   10   9   8   7   6   5   4   3

Human Kinetics
Web site: http://www.humankinetics.com/

United States: Human Kinetics
P.O. Box 5076
Champaign, IL 61825-5076
1-800-747-4457
e-mail: humank@hkusa.com

Canada: Human Kinetics, Box 24040
Windsor, ON N8Y 4Y9
1-800-465-7301 (in Canada only)
e-mail: humank@hkcanada.com

Europe: Human Kinetics, P.O. Box IW14
Leeds LS16 6TR, United Kingdom
(44) 1132 781708
e-mail: humank@hkeurope.com

Australia: Human Kinetics
57A Price Avenue
Lower Mitcham, South Australia 5062
(088) 277 1555
e-mail: humank@hkaustralia.com

New Zealand: Human Kinetics
P.O. Box 105-231, Auckland 1
(09) 523 3462
e-mail: humank@hknewz.com

To my Mom and Dad, Shirley and Bill Twist. I am always very keenly aware that any successes I may enjoy, whether personal relationships or career achievements, all stem from growing up in an incredibly positive and supportive family environment. Because they are such outstanding people and outstanding parents, I am forever indebted to them for the person I am, for the life I have lived, for the life I enjoy today, and for the future I look forward to with great enthusiasm. I am proud to call them my parents and lucky to call them my friends.

To Julie, my favorite person in the world, for making every day a blast, for making life so incredibly fulfilling, for being the most important part of my life, and for being my soulmate and true partner in life.

This book is for the altruistically motivated coaches who are always trying to learn and improve, simply for the benefit of their athletes.

CONTENTS

FOREWORD

What does it take to be a top hockey player? Certainly stickhandling, passing, and shooting skills are essential. A tough mental attitude is also required. But what's just as important is proper physical conditioning.

Hockey talent needs to be supported by a complete conditioning program. That's how a player reaches the highest levels of performance over the course of a season or career. It doesn't matter how talented you are—if you don't work hard at conditioning, you won't reach your true potential. To be a great player you have to combine talent and hard work and be dedicated to your preparation.

You'll find the total training package in *Complete Conditioning for Ice Hockey*. This book will help you work on your weaknesses and build on your strengths. It's the best guide for getting faster, stronger, more agile, and more powerful.

I recommend this book based on first-hand experience. You see, author Pete Twist is our team's strength and conditioning coach. He helps young players develop the physical tools they need to succeed at the NHL level, and he helps top players improve and reach a new level. And he coached me on the ice and worked with me off the ice after my knee was injured, helping me get back into game condition.

Coach Twist's program is based on solid research in strength and conditioning. But what makes it special is that it's applied specifically to hockey. The book will improve your skating, hockey abilities, and competitive performance—not only give you larger muscles and more endurance.

Pete has the coaching expertise and the hockey skills to run both effective and enjoyable on-ice practices. His off-ice exercises and drills are designed to meet the demands of games and to build the physical tools each skill will draw on.

Another plus about Pete's program is that the variety of drills make training more fun. It prevents year-round workouts from becoming old and boring because you are doing different things all the time. Yet, you can see that each activity or exercise has a purpose and how it will benefit your game.

Hockey coaches can teach basic skills to young players, but NHL-level skills, mental and visual skills, and on-ice awareness come more naturally. Everyone starts out with different levels of natural talent. But with specific conditioning, you can improve to the next level and get the most out of your talent. I wouldn't score as many goals if I didn't work hard at conditioning. Likewise, I wouldn't skate as well without specific conditioning.

The best part is that conditioning is easy. Of course it's very hard work, but I call it the easiest part because it is something everyone is capable of doing. All players at all levels can improve their game with *Complete Conditioning for Ice Hockey*. It's sure to have a positive impact on your game.

—Pavel Bure, Vancouver Canucks

ACKNOWLEDGMENTS

I'd like to recognize the Vancouver Canucks Hockey Club and Orca Bay Sports & Entertainment for their generous support of the educational process and their genuine interest in improving the opportunities for young hockey players.

The following four people provided both their time and expertise to review the manuscript's first draft: Lorne Goldenberg and George Nevole Jr. reviewed the sport science and coaching content; Dr. Sue Crawford reviewed the nutrition chapter; and Julie Rogers reviewed the exercise science material and exercise technique instructions.

I'd like to acknowledge Steve Larmer for his long-term support of this project. All players in this book offer good examples of the attributes one aims to develop through conditioning, and they are representative of the positive attitude, commitment, and coachability players need to reach for their absolute best. The coaches give you an idea of the importance of being progressive, open minded, embracing change, and incorporating the sport sciences into the coaching process. The following coaches and players deserve recognition for their interest in helping educate the hockey community: Trevor Linden, Tim Hunter, Bret Hedican, Dave Babych, Jyrki Lumme, Mike Peca, Martin Gelinas, Gino Odjick, Pavel Bure, Jeff Brown, Geoff Courtnall, Alek Stojanov, and Corey Hirsch, who appear in exercise and drill photographs.

Thanks to Steve Larmer, Pavel Bure, Tim Hunter, Paul Coffey, Curt Fraser, Don Cherry, Murray Craven, Pat Quinn, Jyrki Lumme, Bret Hedican, Joe Sakic, Chris Chelios, Jeremy Roenick, Wayne Gretzky, Doug Gilmour, Geoff Courtnall, Keith Brown, George Nevole, Lorne Goldenberg, and Sue Crawford, who shared their experience and offered tips, advise, and philosophies on conditioning for the benefit of readers; Bob Gainey, John Vanbiesbrouck, Jim Gregory, Wally Harris, Mike Gartner, Jose Charbonneau, Wayne Bonney, Kay Whitmore, Mike Peca, Dean Chynoweth, Mike Keenan, and Gordie Hurlbert, who generously shared valuable ideas in interviews that, due to space limitations, were not included in this book. Instead, they will appear in the *Journal of Hockey Conditioning and Player Development*.

This book, from the initial manuscript, several drafts, through to the final copy, was written with the only spare time I had—from11:00 P.M. to 7:00 A.M. So I would be remiss if I didn't thank my partner in life, Julie Rogers, not only for her support, but also for her patience as I dedicated endless evenings and entire nights to the demands of this project, sacrificing valuable family time to see this through to fruition. And our dog Rico, for staying up all night with me on several dozen occasions, and the 4:30 A.M. tug of war games up on our roof deck for good writing breaks. I'd also like to thank The Doors, CCR, Van Morrison, B.B. King, and April Wine for helping me make it through the all-night writing sessions.

I am thankful to McMaster University, University of British Columbia, and the National Strength and Conditioning Association for many sport science and coaching educational opportunities; and to Rick Ley, Glen Hanlon, Stan Smyl, Pat Quinn, George McPhee, Jack McIlhargey, Steve Tambellini, Mike Penny, Curt Fraser, and Ron Smith for sharing their philosophies on player development.

I am indebted to Human Kinetics' Ted Miller and Kirby Mittelmeier for transforming my words and ideas into this book. Still others deserve many thanks: Carlos Mascarenhas, Jack Murray, Dr. Ted Rhodes, Dusan Benicky, Devin Smith, Norm Jewison, Veronica Varhaug, Sonya Lumholst-Smith, Mark Kling, Ric Thomsen, Bob Dunn, Doug Cole, Michael Reynolds, Al Hemsworth, Dan Gibbons, Howard Hemper, Fred Garvin MP, Dr. McGillicuddy, Dr. Ben Dover, Pat Park, Rick Minch, Barry Watkins, Greg Bouris, John Wharton, David Patriquin, and Kent Kallberg.

Last, and most important, I would like to recognize the late Larry Ashley. I had the privilege of working with Larry, who held the position of chief medical trainer for the Vancouver Canucks from 1981 to 1995. Within the hockey community, Larry is known as a pioneer in the fields of medical training, rehabilitation, and physiological testing. Larry was instrumental in forming the Professional Hockey Athletic Trainers Association and also served as its president. Larry not only raised the quality of medical care in hockey, but also set the standards for ethical medical practice.

Larry Ashley will be long-remembered for initiating many progressive changes in hockey, his commitment to the sport and his athletes, and his love of the game. The world of hockey is indebted to the ingenuity and dedication of Larry Ashley, who easily validated his reputation as hockey's top trainer.

Above and beyond all of his accomplishments, Ash was truly a good man.

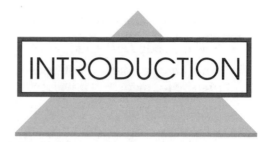

INTRODUCTION

Hockey is a sport of complex motor skills within an environment of explosive speed and intense physical contact. The game demands large muscle mass and exceptional strength for aggressive body contact, but also a very lean body mass for explosive power, efficient movement, and high-speed agility. Skating itself is an unnatural movement for the human body. Add carrying a stick, controlling a puck, reacting to a constantly changing environment, delivering and receiving bodychecks, going all-out for 45 seconds and then sitting down and resting, plus continually stopping and starting and changing directions, and you have the unique game of hockey. To play this demanding game well requires equally unique and detailed preparation.

I have been contacted by hundreds of coaches and athletes from all over North America and beyond requesting information about conditioning for hockey. My response to all their questions is this book, which I hope provides the guidance needed to understand the sometimes complex domain of hockey conditioning. Here I have analyzed the physiological, bioenergetic, anatomical, biomechanical, neuromuscular, and nutritional demands of ice hockey, cutting through the jungle of theoretical information to provide only the practicalities a coach or athlete must know to improve hockey skills, technique, and game performance. From my inventory of over two thousand off-ice and on-ice exercises and drills, I have selected those that are most specific to ice hockey and easiest to use with players.

The information offered here is meant for young and old, rookie and veteran, and both recreational and professional athletes; what you'll learn will help you ensure safe and effective conditioning, optimize athletic abilities, improve sport performance, and reduce injuries. The ultimate goal, of course, is to help players achieve their greatest level of potential while remaining injury free and healthy.

By reading this book, you'll learn

- how the body works and how it responds to different stressors,
- what kinds of demands hockey places on the body and how to prepare for them,
- how physiological components affect skill execution,
- what to improve and how to improve it, and
- how to tie together all the physical attributes needed for hockey at different times of the season.

Hockey is one of the most complex sports in the world, and its physical demands reflect this. Hockey players do not go through conditioning only to "get in shape"—development requires specific exercise that helps players acquire skills and improve game performance. Conditioning is structured to help the player skate, shoot, pass, check, stop and start, pivot, take one-on-ones, cross over, play at a higher intensity, go harder for longer into a shift, and recover faster between shifts on the bench.

Conditioning programs from other sports will not prepare a player for a hockey game. Some have mistakenly turned to speedskating programs for hockey preparation, since they both take place on ice, and speedskating involves "speed." But even speedskating conditioning is unsuitable for hockey, and comparing the two sports illustrates why. Speedskating involves continual forward skating around a track, building up to a top speed, and then trying to maintain that top speed over the entire distance. Speedskating does not involve carrying a stick, handling a puck, passing, shooting, bodychecking, dropping to block shots, warding off opponents, stops and starts, continual switching between decelerating and accelerating, backward skating, lateral movement, pivots, and constant changes in direction. Unless the player can hop over the boards for a line change and skate one full lap of the ice before entering the play, how does speedskating fit in? This is not to belittle speedskating as a sport, but the comparison of it to hockey exemplifies why hockey requires a specific conditioning program. Each sport has its own unique characteristics, biomechanical requirements, and specific physiological demands.

In the past 20 years, the game of hockey has changed in many ways. The emphasis and content of coaching is different. Player involvement is different. Players are bigger, faster, quicker, and stronger than they used to be. As the game has changed, so has the preparation. Explains Curt Fraser, a 12-year NHL veteran with Chicago, Vancouver, and

Minnesota: "The year I started playing there was a kind of new genera-tion of players who came to camp ready to play from day one. We came to camp in shape, and the older players didn't. They still came expecting to use that first month to get ready. So we started out way ahead of them, and that's probably what helped us make the team and enjoy a fairly good first season."

Not only have the game and the athletes changed, so too has the schedule. Players at all levels face a heavier game schedule. The NHL schedule, when you count exhibition games, regular-season games, and possible playoff games, includes over a hundred games a year. The off-season is almost a month shorter than basketball's, $1\frac{1}{2}$ months shorter than baseball's, and less than half that of football's. Conditioning is no longer a big advantage for a player—it is an absolute necessity. To build competitive teams, coaches must learn how conditioning affects game performance and skill acquisition; they must know what to focus on and when to focus on it. Of course players too must make the commitment.

Unfortunately, many hockey players have been taught skills and techniques independent of the physical attributes necessary to perform them. For those coaches who understood the need for strength and conditioning, educational resources did not exist. They read books on skills, systems and tactics, and lots of Xs and Os, but there was nothing out there to educate them on hockey conditioning.

With the help of state and national programs and seminars offering educational opportunities and certifications, hockey coaches have pro-gressed to a point where all agree that players need to be in shape to play the game well. Many have even progressed to the point where they know that players must be conditioned *specifically* for hockey. Still, conditioning is often separated from skill learning.

Skill improvement and conditioning are interweaved closer than most coaches and players realize. Not only are certain physical attributes needed as a base for skill acquisition, but skill and conditioning actually complement each other. The skating stride is a good example. A player who is a technically sound skater is a mechanically efficient skater, using less energy and delaying fatigue, while poor skaters use up a lot more energy, leading to quicker fatigue. A well-conditioned player will be able to skate longer without the fatigue that adversely affects skating technique, while poorly conditioned athletes will tire quicker, affecting their technique. Acquiring proper skating technique also requires a base of strength, flexibility, speed, quickness, and agility. A strength imbal-ance inhibits technique, and lack of flexibility interferes with complex skating patterns. Skill and technique acquisition or improvement must be integrated with conditioning for optimal player development.

In a team sport, it is easy to get away from individual player development. This is especially true in a multidimensional sport like hockey, where coaches spend a lot of time coaching team situations and preparing for opponents, teaching things like breakouts, power-play systems, three-on-twos, and so on. But for players to fulfill their unique, individual potentials, they need to be developed *as individuals*. The commitment rests on the player's shoulders as well as the coach's. Many things are outside a player's control—a coach's evaluation, for instance, or some skills and abilities that seem to come more naturally to some than to others—but five factors are always in the player's control: work ethic, mental preparation, positioning, choice of diet, and conditioning. The best players understand they have this control and they exercise it—and by doing so they sometimes far surpass those with more "natural gifts" but who do not work as hard or prepare as well.

Coaches must stay tuned in to their players' individual development needs. For today's coaches of youth hockey, this not only includes hockey development but also general athletic development. There are several reasons for this. One is that many young players have been pushed early on into specializing in hockey, at the expense of participating in other sports. As a result, they lack a good base of athleticism. Compounding this problem is the fact that many schools are cutting back on their physical education courses, eliminating activities.

Also, as children spend more time in front of TVs and video games, and more parents drive their children to school, youths are becoming more sedentary. This lifestyle is often made worse by a diet of junk food. Kids are left with poor fitness and poor health. Today, half the 12-year-olds in North America have at least one symptom of heart disease! The bottom line is that many youngsters are not active enough and are not participating in a variety of activities, which creates a greater need to spend extra time on practicing general movement patterns to develop balance, coordination, agility, and basic athletic abilities.

I commend all the coaches who have contacted me to ask for conditioning information. They want to expand their coaching repertoire and have a sincere concern for their players' development. I also thank coaches who are reading this book. Your athletes are a fortunate bunch. In our society, 20 percent of the people do 80 percent of the work, and they achieve 80 percent of the accomplishments. Clearly, you are among the 20 percent willing to put in the extra effort it takes to improve.

The same can be said for you athletes driven enough to improve as hockey players that you pick up this book to check out the exercises and drills you can work on independently. Your motivation is to be admired, and you'll see that it pays off in the long run. Yours is the smart approach.

You need specific conditioning, quality versus quantity, intensity versus volume.

Before you proceed further into the book, I want to stress at the outset that weight training makes up less than 10 percent of my conditioning programs. It's true that improved strength, increased lean muscle mass, increased power, and improved muscular endurance can all come from weight training. But while weight training can help hockey performance, it will only be a benefit when it's used specifically to make a better *hockey* player—not a powerlifter or bodybuilder or weightlifter. Weight training comprises just one part of preparing an athlete for hockey.

Complete conditioning for hockey is a multidimensional program. This book addresses all of the key components that I prescribe for hockey players. My on-ice and off-ice practices develop aerobic power, the anaerobic energy systems, lactic acid toleration, muscular power, muscular endurance, rotational strength, hockey-specific strength, speed, agility, quick feet, quick hands, static and dynamic flexibility, and, of course, technique. Developing a base of strength and lean muscle mass; improving body composition; integrating warm-ups, postgame recovery, and nutrition; plus preventing and rehabilitating injuries are also key parts of the player's complete conditioning program.

Before utilizing this book, there is something I'd like you to consider for your coaching philosophy. Unfortunately, minor sport is plagued with coaches who use physical activity as a consequence of poor play and skill execution errors. Often players are commanded to skate lines or do push ups after a loss as a form of disciplinary action. I am definitely an advocate of hard work, but I am unequivocally against using conditioning as a punishment. Conditioning should be used positively because it is designed to help players improve and prepare for competition. The purpose of conditioning is to help players develop, which any player motivated to improve should be enthusiastic about. But I don't know anyone who would take the initiative to participate in an activity that has been commonly presented as punishment. This will not only affect short term athletic development and limit potential, but will also produce lifelong negative perceptions of fitness and wellness activities. Use conditioning constructively and present it for what it is—an opportunity for individuals and teams to prepare and improve.

Key to Diagrams

X	Player
△	Cones (pylons)
●	Puck
᠑	Goal net
⟶	Forward skating
- - - ➤	Backward skating
—·—➤	Passing
·········➤	Lateral crossovers

CHAPTER 1

FITNESS BASICS FOR HOCKEY

The two-phase process to building fitness for hockey includes (1) improving general fitness, or getting "in shape," and (2) hockey-specific conditioning. Getting in shape means improving aerobic power, flexibility, strength, and diet while decreasing body fat and increasing muscle mass. This kind of general fitness is important to overall health and will usually help you perform almost any activity a little better. For hockey players, improved aerobic power aids endurance, decreased body fat allows for faster, more efficient skating, and added strength and flexibility and a healthy diet help you maintain your exercise regimen with reduced risk of injury.

The second phase of building fitness for hockey requires conditioning *specifically* for the demands you'll encounter on the ice. Exercises and drills must be selected and completed with specific exercise prescriptions so that the players' physical and physiological development best suits the game of ice hockey. Sometimes gains in strength, flexibility, or lean body mass can actually detract from hockey skills, because the "improvements" are not appropriate for the demands of hockey. Meanwhile, other development crucial to hockey success is sometimes overlooked. The anaerobic energy system needs to be conditioned, as players depend on this system for explosive movements and intense action. Equally important are quickness and agility, which need to be developed for improved reaction time, coordination, footwork, and explosiveness. Muscular endurance and power are also essential to help improve skills and game performance and to allow players to perform longer before fatigue deters proper execution.

Hockey players should first develop general fitness to obtain a good base of conditioning before moving on to developing sport-specific physical attributes. Once general fitness has been attained, there are a few important guidelines as to which specific area to develop first. Because the aerobic energy system helps the body recover from bouts of anaerobic activity, it's necesssary to develop the aerobic system first. Similarly, proper strength, lean mass, and flexibility development is required before progressing to work on muscular endurance, power, speed, quickness, and agility.

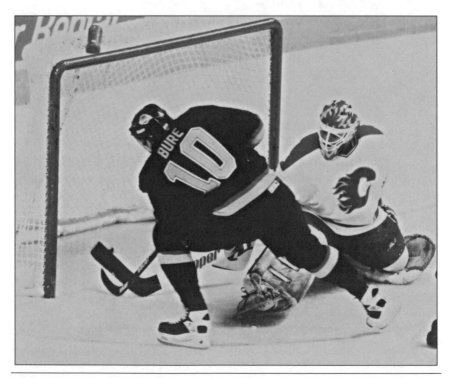

Pavel Bure lunges to the left to score a double-overtime playoff goal against the Calgary Flames.

PRINCIPLES OF CONDITIONING

Several training variables can be manipulated to make a conditioning program optimally beneficial. One general priniciple to remember is to always stress quality over quantity. Long, general workouts with random exercises do little to improve conditioning or on-ice abilities. A short, intense, specific workout produces much greater results. Other important principles for hockey conditioning involve safety, exercise preparation, progressive overload, rest and recovery, periodization, and specificity. Considerations for each of these areas will be detailed in the following sections. These principles help coaches structure practices and are manipulated to present further challenges for players as they improve.

Safety Considerations

Conditioning builds your body up. Hockey tears your body down. More conditioning helps repair your body and build it back up again. Then comes the next hockey game . . . it is a constant cycle. But tearing down the body should be restricted to hockey itself—the on-ice and off-ice conditioning you do to prepare for hockey should never be the *cause* of injury. So, when developing a conditioning program, always think "safety first." Follow these guidelines:

- Establish an adequate base of strength, aerobic fitness, and athleticism before progressing to intense or explosive exercises and complex movements.
- Always assess technique. Technique includes body position, balance, foot placement, amount of knee bend, and landing position. Technique corrections help prevent injury and optimize fitness and performance.
- Warm up before each and every workout.
- Use a break-in period when starting a new conditioning program or when introducing new components (e.g., plyometrics) to an existing program.
- Always rest each body part after a vigorous workout, allowing 24 to 48 hours rest and recovery.
- For off-ice conditioning, wear footwear that provides lateral support and good shock absorption. Wear crosstrainers or high-tops when performing plyometrics and agility drills.

- For all heavy weight training, a spotter should be present to assess technique, help move the weight into starting position, and, if necessary, assist with the last couple of reps.
- Make sure that all surfaces are clean and that all unnecessary equipment and nonparticipating athletes are clear of the area.
- Drink plenty of water before, during, and after workouts, especially in hot weather.

Exercise Preparation

Warm up and stretch before each workout. An ideal warm-up consists of light, low-impact cardiovascular exercise for about 5 to 10 minutes at 60 to 70 percent maximum heart rate. "Breaking a sweat" indicates a sufficient warm-up. A good warm-up raises core muscle temperature (which increases muscle elasticity), increases the rate of agonist muscle contraction, and increases the rate of antagonist muscle relaxation. (Agonist muscles contract to contribute to the movement; antagonist muscles oppose the agonist muscles and must relax to allow movement.)

Following a warm-up, complete the preparation routine with stretching; this will increase muscle relaxation, elasticity, and extensibility. Regular, long-term stretching will increase the range of motion across each joint. Improper stretching can result in minor muscle tears and decreased flexibility. For beneficial stretching, move into each stretch slowly and smoothly, and hold in a comfortable position for 30 to 60 seconds, without bouncing or jerking. If there is not enough time to adequately warm up and properly stretch, you should use gentle, fluid dynamic stretching to prepare for activity. Dynamic stretching will warm up the muscles and lubricate the joints. See chapter 2 for more on flexibility.

Break-In Period

Muscles require time to adapt to new loads imposed on the body. When starting or restarting any conditioning program, begin with a break-in period. During this period (about two weeks), initiate your program with light weights, low intensities, and low speeds. When starting a new conditioning program, detrained muscles are susceptible to injury during contraction. A break-in period allows safe, sensible progression to the eventual training level.

Using muscles unaccustomed to weight training and conditioning will produce a delayed muscle soreness. If they do too much too soon, players will be quite stiff and sore 24 to 48 hours after a new workout.

Steve Larmer

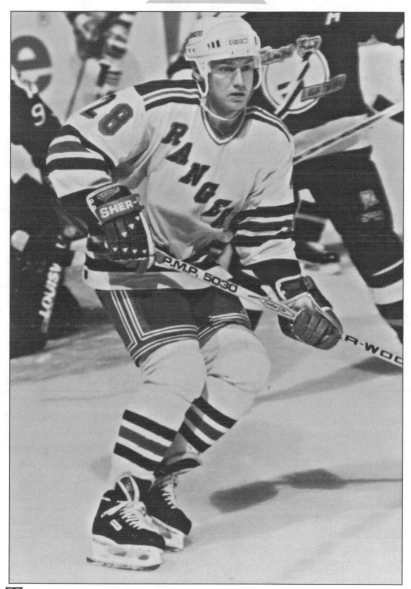

Throughout a long, successful career characterized by consistency and durability, Steve Larmer demonstrated both offensive playmaking and scoring abilities along with a defensive commitment and willingness for physical play. From the NHL Rookie of the Year Award in 1982-83 with the Chicago Black Hawks, leading all rookies in scoring (will 43 goals and 47 assists) and finishing a plus 44 the same year, scoring 20-plus goals a year for 13 consecutive seasons, making the All-Star teams in 1990 and 1991, to being named hockey's "Man of the Year" by the *Hockey News* and by *Inside Hockey* in 1990-91, Larmer quietly compiled an impressive list of individual accomplishments. His contribution to team success is highlighted by a 1991 Canada Cup championship for Team Canada (scoring the series winning goal) and a 1994 Stanley Cup Championship with the New York Rangers.

From day one to present day, Larmer notices many distinct changes in the game. "In my first year, training camp was for getting into shape. Only a very small percentage of players did any off-ice workouts in the summer. Now it's the other way around— at least 95 percent of the players are doing all of their hard workouts in the summertime, getting ready for training camp. The mindset of everybody has changed in the last 5 or 6 years. With an 84-game schedule plus travel, if you don't prepare in the summer, there's no way you can get ahead during the hockey season. If someone comes into training camp and they're not in shape, it really shows up. They are behind the eight ball all year. There's no way they're going to catch up."

Larmer played more than 1,000 NHL games, scoring over 1,000 points. He played in 884 consecutive games, the third longest Iron Man streak in NHL history, lasting 11 years from 1982 through to 1993. The secret to career longevity? "A physically fit athlete is less prone to injury, and if you are mentally prepared to play a game your chances of getting hurt are much less. I always tried to be aware of what was going on around me, what *all* the other players were doing. Never let up for a second, play hard through everything, don't take it easy, while always expecting the unexpected— from the very start of a shift until the very end of the shift. Lifestyle habits are important too. Taking care of yourself, eating right, proper nutrition, getting the right amount of sleep and rest, plus physically working out all go hand in hand."

Steve's advice for minor hockey players? "When you're young you should play more than one sport. Playing all different sports helps conditioning and athletic development. Baseball is a great sport for hand-eye coordination. Lacrosse is great for learning how to take a hit and learning how to roll off checks. Complement these sports with a well-rounded, varied conditioning program."

Even world-class athletes experience delayed muscle soreness if they work out after a layoff of just a few weeks. Overworking deconditioned muscles will slow down progression because the athlete will miss workouts due to stiffness and soreness.

Even if participating in a regular, intense conditioning program that consists, for example, of aerobic, anaerobic, strength, and flexibility components, an athlete should still use a break-in period when introducing new components (e.g., speed or plyometrics) to the program. A break-in period also allows time to learn the proper technique and movements with lower risk of injury.

Progressive Overload

Exercise must be stressful enough to stimulate a physical change in the body. Often this involves working muscles and energy systems against a heavy enough resistance to induce momentary fatigue (overloading). Training sets the muscles and body parts up so they will adapt and recover to become stronger and more fit.

As improvements are made, the conditioning program must progress to keep challenging the muscles and energy systems. The basic exercise variables manipulated to progress your program and promote further physical development include training volume, density, intensity, frequency, and duration. Ongoing physical adaptations depend on *progressive overload* to ensure the training stimulus is stressful enough to challenge the body. You may accomplish this by increasing the number of sprint repetitions (volume), decreasing rest intervals for bike sprints (density), cycling with a higher heart rate (intensity), progressing from three to four strength-training workouts per week (frequency), or running for a longer amount of time (duration).

Volume

Volume refers to the total number of sets and reps in your program. Volume is often quantified as sets × reps × load for a given workout. A higher training volume often produces better training results; however, volume is manipulated at different times of the season to achieve specific conditioning results. A large training volume is used to build a base of conditioning, specifically improving strength and lean mass, decreasing fat, and sometimes improving aerobic fitness. Lower volumes are characteristic of high-intensity training that includes anaerobic power and capacity, speed, quickness, and agility. Lower volumes are also common during the in-season period to accommodate games, on-ice practices, and travel.

Density

Workout *density* involves the amount of rest between sets. Circuit training would be an example of a dense workout with little or no rest between exercises. A high-density workout usually features a lower duration and volume and is therefore more time-efficient. High-density workouts are sometimes used in-season, when fitting in a dry-land strength and muscular endurance workout, often postgame.

Intensity

Intensity is a measure of physical exertion and is the most important factor in physical adaptation—the more intense the training, the greater the physical change in your body. When strength training, lifting to momentary fatigue each set will produce greater changes in the body. For aerobic activity, raising your heart rate to within a certain training zone will result in the desired cardiovascular changes. To adhere to the progressive overload principle, it is most time-efficient to increase intensity.

Frequency

Frequency—that is, the number of times you train—also affects conditioning. For substantial physical changes, training must be performed three or more times weekly. Maintaining a certain fitness level requires at least one or two training sessions per week, depending on the level.

Duration

For a given intensity, the greater the *duration* of training, the greater the training effect. The duration can be manipulated to satisfy the progressive overload principle. Common examples include lengthening the time of a jog or cycling workout. But the length of time an athlete should work out each session depends on the type of training. Remember that quality training is much more efficient and beneficial than sheer quantity training.

Rest and Recovery

The stimulus to a training effect is the training session itself; however, the actual physical improvement, or physical adaptation, occurs *after* the training session is over. Microscopic muscle tears occur naturally during an intense workout. The muscles need time to adapt to training loads as they repair and grow to a new level. The muscle groups worked need 24 to 48 hours to recover from a training session. During this period

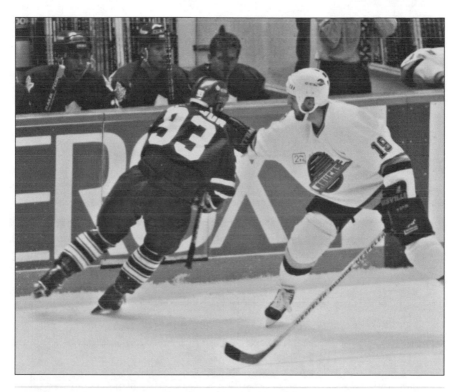

Tim Hunter uses upper strength from lateral raises and upright rows (see chapter 4) to ward off and contain his opponent.

of rest, the muscle responds to the training stimulus and physical development occurs.

The rest and recovery period is as important to conditioning gains as the actual workout itself. If an adequate rest period is not taken, over-training will cause an injury and physical development will be delayed. As Keith Brown, a 16-year NHL veteran with Chicago and Florida, explains, "When I was young I used to train too hard. I'd overtrain, tear my body down, and become more susceptible to injuries. Now, even if I still have lots of energy after working out, I realize I should take time off to rest. I feel so much better, and I end up more fit and stronger."

Many coaches still have trouble with the "rest" concept. Teams have been known to practice every single day, simply because that's the way it's always been done or because they are worried that they need to look like they are working hard to improve. Because hockey is rooted in tradition, the hockey community has often resisted change. Today, many coaches and players are beginning to understand that improvement relies on physical recovery, and that both players and teams benefit from mental and emotional rest.

Wayne Gretzky

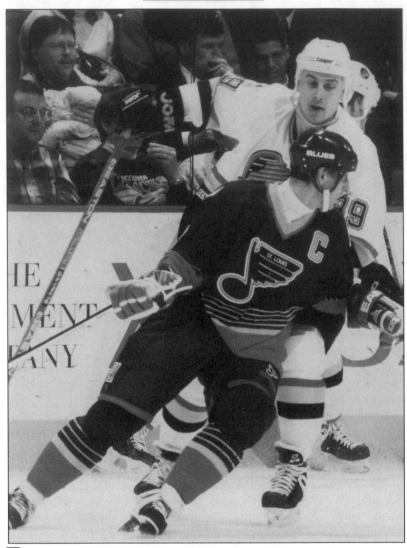

Recently acquired by the New York Rangers, Wayne Gretzky has won nine Hart Memorial Trophies (NHL MVP). Five Lester B. Pearson Awards (NHL outstanding player, selected by players). Ten Art Ross Trophies (scoring championship). Four Lady Byng Memorial Trophies for most gentlemanly player. Four Stanley Cup Championships. Fifteeen NHL All-Star games . . . the list goes on. Gretzky's long, ultrasuccessful career over 17 NHL seasons playing 1,253 games and accumulating 2,585 points, has resulted in his owning or sharing 61 NHL records. Year after year of withstanding the rigors of the NHL schedule, the physical contact, the competitive challenge, he still has the endurance to play 30-plus minutes a game.

About the role conditioning plays for the highest skilled players, Gretzky explains, "Even the most skilled players can benefit from conditioning. Besides improving physical performance parameters and supporting skill execution, there are other benefits to on-ice performance. For a better conditioned athlete, there is less chance of injury, and conditioning promotes *career* longevity. The player also becomes mentally stronger, after enduring the intense efforts required for conditioning and staying dedicated toward preparing and improving." However, conditioning did not used to be a part of most players' hockey routine. "Originally, only a handful of players worked out in the off-season. Today, there's a high level of conditioning in the off-season. Almost all of the players work out both on-ice and off-ice."

As the NHL's all-time leading scorer, what advice would Gretzky have for a young, aspiring player hopeful of future scoring feats? Repetitively practicing shooting? No—just the opposite. For young athletes, Gretzky recommends, "that they do not focus on one sport. Kids should play all sports. Varied sport participation will help their hand-eye coordination and improve their overall conditioning and athleticism. Team sports, at a young age, also help them learn to be unselfish." And there is no one of such great individual accomplishment more unselfish than Gretzky.

Periodization

Periodization, or the schedule and design of your conditioning program, divides the year into different cycles to help organize conditioning programs. Periodization is based on scientific principles that suggest the best time and best method for conditioning.

During the season, periodization accommodates game and travel schedules to make time for workouts with adequate rest and recovery. Training volume, density, intensity, frequency, and duration can be manipulated to control the training effect. Variables such as speed of movement and movement patterns can also be adjusted. Drills can be selected to prescribe exercise suitable to each individual and the time of season.

The hockey year is divided into four phases—the off-season, pre-season, in-season, and postseason. What is conditioned and how it is conditioned will vary depending on the phase. See chapter 8, "Conditioning for Every Season," for details.

Specificity

Some players dedicate a lot of time and effort to general workouts, hoping they can later benefit from this nonspecific training during hockey-specific actions. But any benefits from general workouts will not transfer to the ice. Often, nonspecific training is actually counterproductive.

Training mainly with exercises nonspecific in movement pattern, speed of movement, range of movement, joint angles, contraction type, and contraction force will hinder on-ice skill execution that requires very different movement patterns, speeds of movement, ranges of movement, joint angles, contraction types, and contraction forces. My specificity principle also considers muscle groups used, work times, distances, and rest periods. The more specific the conditioning program is to game demands, the more the training effects will transfer onto the ice to benefit skills and improve hockey performance. Hockey Lunges and Speedtraxx Strides are good examples of sport-specific resistance training exercises that prepare athletes for on-ice activity because they use all the "skating muscles" and incorporate a similar movement pattern.

ADJUNCTS TO CONDITIONING

Other factors important to developing a sound conditioning program include tracking players' progress and optimizing nutritional choices and timing of meals.

Testing and Recording

Recording the results of conditioning sessions ensures proper monitoring and refinement of players' programs and shows the progression made toward goals. Consider keeping a conditioning log book in which you list the results of on-ice and off-ice conditioning sessions. Record the date, type of exercise (e.g., strength), muscle group being worked, name of exercise, weight lifted, number of sets and reps, rest times between sets, and total workout duration. For aerobic activity, record peak and average heart rates, distance, and the speed or level (e.g., level 8 on a stair-climbing machine). On-ice conditioning may target several components within one practice, so you also should record drills, drill diagrams, what they are intended to work on, and which players participated. To help design future practices, add useful information to quantify the structure and result of the session—for example, work and rest interval times, heart rates, and subjective feedback (e.g., "my legs were really tight and tired after that drill").

The more quantifiable details you record, the more accurately you can assess conditioning and learning. A consistent workout log allows you to monitor and adjust training, as necessary, to help ensure that players are not overtraining or undertraining. The log will also help regulate a continual upward adjustment for steady progress.

For the past decade, Dr. Ted Rhodes and Dusan Benicky of the University of British Columbia have been overseeing the Canucks' physiological testing, implementing tests for aerobic power, anaerobic power and capacity, strength, flexibility, and body fat. We also use on-ice tests for quickness and agility. The results of the physiological tests are used, along with coach evaluations, when designing individualized programs for players. See chapter 8 for more testing information.

Nutrition

Nutrition is a key link between preparation and performance. Optimal nutrition supplies energy for conditioning, allows for more intense training, delays fatigue, and helps keep you healthy and well. Proper nutrition also aids faster and more complete recovery after workouts, so players will have a full energy supply for the next practice and be able to practice more frequently. Eating the right things at the right times helps to produce superior physical and physiological results from workouts. In chapter 7, I show you how to make the right food choices and how to time meals to maximize performance.

CHAPTER 2

FLEXIBILITY

Your body is constructed of over 600 muscles and 206 bones. The muscles are attached to the bones by your tendons. Each of your muscles crosses over a specific joint in a way that causes the bones of that joint to move when the muscle contracts (shortens). For example, your biceps muscle attaches to a bone on your upper arm, crosses your elbow joint, and then inserts on the bone of your lower arm. When you contract your biceps (bend your arm at the elbow), the muscle shortens and pulls up your lower arm. This is the way your body moves: Your muscles tell your bones what to do.

For smooth, coordinated movement on the ice, your muscles need to contract and relax at just the right time. Stretching your muscles before practice or a game will improve your flexibility and prepare your muscles for the range of movement hockey demands. A warmed, stretched muscle is elastic and extensible and will contract and relax quickly. A cold, unstretched muscle restricts movement and is easily injured. A quick movement of a cold muscle can result in a muscle tear or strain. Because movements in hockey are so unpredictable, with players constantly reacting to sudden changes on the ice, your muscles should be able to move easily through all possible motions—even those unexpected movements you make when you receive a hit or fall from an awkward position. A regular stretching program increases the extensibility of muscles, improves the range of motion around joints, and reduces the risk and severity of injury.

A warm-up and stretching routine before each practice and game can also help you mentally—it might be the best time to relax and focus on the game ahead.

Stretching before activity is essential for immediate gains in flexibility and safety, but the best time to stretch for long-term gains in flexibility is *after* a game or practice. Following activity, a muscle's temperature is at its highest, allowing for easier stretching. Stretching after activity also reduces delayed muscle soreness and helps your muscles recover from exercise.

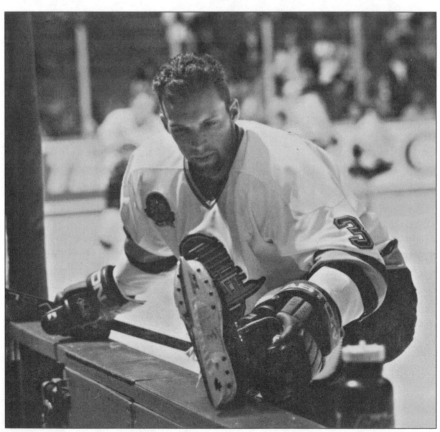

Bret Hedican stretches before a game.

A common myth holds that strength and lean muscle mass gains decrease flexibility. This misconception has probably resulted from coaches who witnessed players who adopted nonspecific weight training. If an athlete's play suffered, it was probably due to a poorly structured strength and conditioning program that was not suitable for the characteristics of hockey, not because strength and muscle gains decreased flexibility. Flexibility at a joint is affected by the degree to which a muscle can be stretched, not by the strength and size of the muscle.

A case in point is Shawn Antoski. At 246 pounds, he's the biggest hockey player I've coached at any level. He had the largest muscle mass of any player on the team and was the second strongest. He was also the fastest and by far the most flexible—even more flexible than our goaltenders.

HOCKEY-SPECIFIC FLEXIBILITY

Areas of the body of special concern to hockey players, when it comes to flexibility, are the hamstrings and the lower back region.

Because skating is a bent-leg activity, few hockey players fully extend their rear leg when pushing off each stride. During the skating stride, the hamstrings are rarely stretched to their full length. Because muscles will shorten when not used to their maximum length, lack of full extension during skating results in tightened hamstrings, which, over time, lead to back injuries or groin pulls. Heightened flexibility at the hips, groin, hamstrings, and thighs will not only prevent injury but also improve skating speed and footwork.

Special preventive attention is needed in the lower back region. Hockey players skate with a slight back flexion, which places demands on lower back strength and flexibility. Without specific preparation, the lower back will not withstand the continual isometric contraction of the back extensors in the skating position or the stressful twisting actions that occur during a game, such as the forceful trunk rotation when shooting. Fighting through checks and warding off opponents also places a lot of stress on the lower back region.

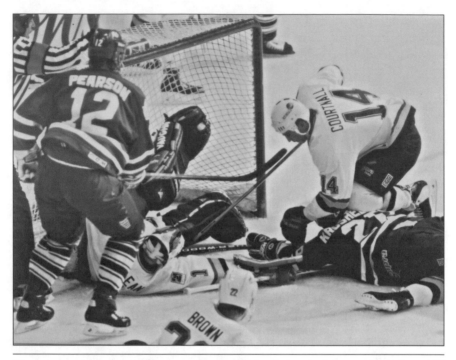

Hockey exposes a player to an endless supply of physical demands during skill execution, body contact, and from continually reacting to 11 other players on the ice.

TYPES OF STRETCHES

To do *static stretching* you select a muscle and gently move across a joint until you feel a comfortable stretch on the muscle. Then you stop and hold that position for a short time. The muscle is being stretched in a *static*, or stationary, position. If you lack flexibility in certain areas, static stretches are great for isolating muscles. They are easier to learn than PNF stretches and safer for you than ballistic stretches.

Dynamic stretching combines a warm-up and stretching routine, using warm-up type movements through slow, smooth, graceful, full ranges of motion. Dynamic stretching involves active, full-body actions using fluid movement that may be specific to hockey movement patterns. They can be done in a stationary standing position or while moving around the ice. Dynamic stretching is valuable when a player doesn't have time to fulfill a proper warm-up and static stretching routine, as it stretches, relaxes, and warms the muscles while also lubricating the joints.

PNF (proprioceptive neuromuscular facilitation) stretching is done with a partner. For a hamstring stretch, the partner moves the athlete's leg to stretch the hamstring. Then the athlete contracts the hamstring, trying to push the leg back down, while the partner resists the movement. As the athlete relaxes the muscle, the partner moves the leg deeper into the stretch. PNF stretching typically uses a stretch, contract, relax, and stretch deeper sequence. PNF is an advanced stretching method with an aggressive approach; as such, it should only be attempted under the guidance of someone well-experienced in PNF.

Ballistic stretching involves light bouncing across a joint. This method is not commonly recommended because the bouncing is picked up by your muscle receptors and causes the muscle under stretch to contract. Ultimately, you end up with quick stretches across a contracted muscle, which can result in muscle tears. Your muscles must stay relaxed for stretching.

Table 2.1   Warm-Up and Stretching Benefits

Warm-Up

- Makes muscles more extensible, allowing them to contract and relax quicker, thus aiding skill execution
- Helps prevent injury for the same reasons
- Prepares muscles for stretching

Stretching

- Prepares muscles for on-ice movements, helping to prevent injury
- Increases flexibility and range of motion, thus aiding agility, speed, quickness, and all complex skating and puck-handling skills
- Done pregame allows players time to think about the challenges ahead
- Done postgame or postpractice aids muscle recovery and prevents delayed muscle soreness
- Done regularly produces good flexibility improvements

A FLEXIBILITY PROGRAM FOR HOCKEY

Some players will not be motivated to warm up and stretch on their own. Other players are willing to stretch, but they don't know how to stretch properly. Still others may be willing and know how, but they arrive at the rink too late, leaving inadequate time to warm up and stretch properly off the ice. A big challenge for coaches is getting *all* their players stretching and stretching properly. The best solution might be to make the warm-up and stretching routine a regular part of the practice plan.

Integrating a Flexibility Program

The NHL labor dispute and ensuing lockout in the fall of 1994 presented a unique problem for coaches facing the need to maintain player conditioning. How the Vancouver Canucks handled the problem offers a good illustration of how a flexibility routine can be successfully integrated into a practice plan.

After the lockout ended early in 1995, the media presented countless features on the risk of injuries when resuming play after that long a period. Compounding the concern was the expectation that a shortened season would heighten the intensity of early games, as players focused immediately on playoff contention. The major concern was "too much, too soon," which inevitably leads to injury for athletes in all sports at all levels.

During the lockout, the Canucks' head coach, Rick Ley, and I discussed injury prevention. Warm-ups, stretching, and cooldowns became a major part of the injury prevention program, along with off-ice and on-ice conditioning, individualizing the preparation needs of players, monitoring practice intensities and player nutrition, and scheduling rest and recovery periods. We did no stretching off-ice, because we wanted to control how "warmed up" the players were before they stretched.

Instead, we encouraged off-ice aerobic warm-ups to start warming up the muscles and lubricating the joints. Coach Ley made room in his practices for easy flow warm-up drills followed by team stretching on the ice. At the end of practice we had cooldown drills to help clear the lactic acid from the players' legs and give the legs time to relax, followed by a *second* team stretch. The team stretched together, before and after the high-intensity portion of Coach Ley's practice.

With Rick's willingness to incorporate this into his practice, he minimized the team's injuries, which resulted in a lower injury occurrence than most other teams that year. The players experienced fewer skating related injuries such as groin pulls, hip flexor, low back, and abdominal injuries.

The strategy used by the Canucks to integrate a flexibility program (see sidebar) can work for teams that are on the ice daily. But with heavy game schedules, there are periods when even NHL teams do not have enough practice time. Of course coaches of minor hockey can't justify spending time on a warm-up and stretching if they only have two 50-minute practices a week. Faced with fewer practices, minor hockey coaches often ask how they can fulfill an adequate warm-up and stretching program when they don't have nearly enough time to practice skills, tactics, and systems.

If players are able to get to the rink early enough, warm-up and flexibility exercises can be accomplished together as a team off the ice. However, many factors may prevent this. Parents' schedules may prevent them from taking their child to the rink early enough. Early morning practice times are another limiting factor.

If there's not enough time to do the static stretching *properly* off-ice, and the coach does not have time on-ice, I recommend eliminating the static stretching portion of the practice. The worst thing a player can do is to step out on the ice and stretch a cold muscle, or hurry through a 3- or 4-minute stretching routine in an effort to fit it in to the practice plan.

In these cases, stress the warm-up portion. Use light flow drills at the beginning of practice to allow the muscles to be warmed and joints lubricated during low-intensity drills. If time is limited and something has to be cut out, warming up is much more important than stretching. This is where dynamic stretching can contribute to the preactivity warm-up routine.

It's best to use a dynamic warm-up routine at the beginning of practice as a way to prepare players for activity, whereas static stretching is best after practice to take advantage of the elevated muscle temperatures. Hockey coaches and players who meet twice a week can best work stretching exercises into their program by using dynamic stretching (on their own and within drills) to begin practice and static stretching to end practice. Dynamic stretching is done on-ice, where it can best prepare players for the task of ice hockey, while static stretching can be done off the ice right after practice so it doesn't use up ice time, and so you have the time to do the stretches properly.

STRETCHING GUIDELINES

Despite all the potential benefits of a warm-up and stretching routine (see table 2.1), many of the players I've coached say they have tried stretching, but their muscles ended up feeling tighter or even strained. I tell them that warming up and stretching didn't cause their discomfort—*improper* warm-up and stretching caused it. To stretch successfully, players must do it correctly. Once players try stretching properly, they are sold on the merits. The following is a list of 10 guidelines for static stretching. It's important for players to follow all of them for successful stretching.

Joe Sakic

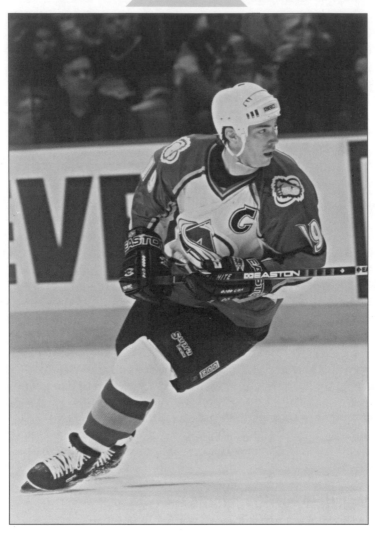

In 1988, Joe Sakic was named the Canadian Major Junior Player of the Year. He was awarded playoff MVP honors and helped the Colorado Avalanche win the Stanley Cup in 1996. Sakic has averaged more than 1.26 points per game. He could always contribute goals and assists, but in between Sakic's junior career and his current status as one of the NHL elite, he has developed into a well-rounded skill player. This can be traced to his conditioning efforts with the Quebec Nordiques.

"As a junior, I trained a bit on weights, but only upper body. No leg work, and no conditioning for things like quickness, agility, or aerobic endurance," explains Sakic. "At my second junior camp I put on a little bit of weight and did not feel great, so from there on I did not train very much. But now I know that this was because I did not train specific for ice hockey."

"In 1991, my third year, I was invited to try out for Team Canada for the Canada Cup Tournament. At the end of camp I was told I needed to improve my leg strength. Going into my fourth year, I met Lorne Goldenberg, coach of conditioning with the Nordiques. Lorne explained to me the importance of developing the legs for hockey, as well as how to train specifically for my sport," Sakic explains, "I worked hard that summer for the first time in my career and as a result of Coach Goldenberg's conditioning program I felt great for the first time in training camp. I was faster and quicker on my feet. I did not feel as fatigued in camp as I had in previous years."

Sakic's development is evident in his six consecutive NHL All-Star team selections and his gold medal in 1994 at the World Championships. "Joe is one of those few highly skilled players who could probably get by on just skill alone," says Goldenberg. But the key is that Sakic doesn't just get by, he tries to get the best performance possible from himself. "Joe's body weight fluctuates between 180 and 185 pounds. He is squatting over 400 pounds, bench pressing over 300 pounds, and is always at the head of the pack in our plyometric tests," says Coach Goldenberg. "It is this combination of strength, speed, and power that allows this small, skilled player to play with the strength of a power forward, and the speed of one of the quickest skaters in the NHL." These attributes, and his overall development, were obvious to everyone following his dominance in the 1996 playoffs.

1. Always warm up a muscle for 5 to 10 minutes prior to stretching. Stretching a cold muscle can cause minor muscular damage and *decreased* flexibility. The warm-up increases the deep core muscle temperature, improving the muscle's elasticity and lubricating the joint.

2. Isolate the muscle to be stretched with very strict technique. Do not "cheat" and alter the exercise slightly just to stretch farther.

3. Move slowly and smoothly through the stretch. Fast movements will cause the muscle to contract (to protect itself). Receptors within your muscles and where they attach to bones can sense the rate of lengthening. If the receptors sense a rapid lengthening, they'll tell the muscle to contract, to protect itself from lengthening too fast.

4. Do not overstretch. Most athletes try to stretch as far as possible, straining to move farther into the stretch. This may seem to make sense, but the receptors in your muscle and at the muscle-tendon attachment also sense *how far* the muscle is being stretched. So straining a joint beyond its range of movement only causes the muscle to contract (to protect itself from being stretched too far). Stretching across a contracted or tight muscle ultimately leads to the formation of inelastic scar tissue. You need to stretch a relaxed muscle, not a contracted muscle. Hold the stretch in a comfortable position. You should feel only a *slight* tension in the muscle, which should subside as you hold the position. If it does not subside, back off to a more relaxed position.

5. Hold the stretch in a static position without bouncing or moving. Remember—stretching a muscle too quickly, bouncing, or holding a stretch as far as you can go causes an involuntary muscle action, which tightens the very muscles you are trying to relax and stretch.

6. Hold each stretch for a minimum of 30 seconds, and optimally up to a minute. The longer you hold an easy stretch, the more likely the muscle will relax and loosen.

7. Inhale before you move into a stretch, exhale as you move into and through the stretch, and then continue to breath normally and freely as you hold the stretch. If a stretched position inhibits your natural breathing pattern, you are obviously not relaxed and are likely straining. Ease up until you can breathe naturally. Take full, relaxed breaths. Never hold your breath.

8. Progress to development stretching. The initial "easy stretch" is designed to help relax the muscle. If your muscle was comfortable during this stretch, you can move another half-inch for a longer stretch. Move farther into the stretch until you again feel a slight tension. The tension should subside. If not, back off to a more comfortable position. Similar to the initial stretch, as you increase the range of motion (progressing deeper into the stretch), exhale slowly.

9. Come out of each stretch as smoothly and slowly as you went into it.

10. Stretch consistently. Regular daily stretching is needed for improvement.

STATIC FLEXIBILITY EXERCISES

T-STRETCH

Focus: Chest

Procedure: Stand in a regular size doorway and place your elbows on the wall, just slightly higher than the shoulders. Place your forearms and hands flat against the wall. Lean into the doorway to stretch the chest muscles.

Duration: Hold stretch for 30 seconds.

On-Ice: If there is plexiglass on both sides, you can use an entrance onto the ice. If not, use one arm at a time where the glass ends at the players' box.

WALL STRETCH

Focus: Shoulders

Procedure: Stand at an angle to a wall. Place one hand up high on the wall and lean your body into the stretch. To advance the stretch, rotate your upper body away from your hand. Repeat for other side.

Duration: Hold stretch for 30 seconds.

On-Ice: Place glove up against plexiglass.

ARM ACROSS BACK STRETCH

Focus: Neck and trapezius

Procedure: Place your right forearm across your lower back. With your left hand, grasp your right hand at the left side of your body. Roll your head to the left and hold for the stretch. Repeat with your left arm across your lower back, rolling your head to the right.

Duration: Hold stretch for 30 seconds.

On-Ice: Same

TRICEPS PULLED ACROSS CHEST STRETCH

Focus: Triceps

Procedure: Stand upright with your knees slightly bent. Place your right arm straight across your chest. With your left hand, pull your right elbow as if trying to move the elbow over your left shoulder. Hold for the stretch. Repeat for other arm.

Duration: Hold stretch for 30 seconds.

On-Ice: Same

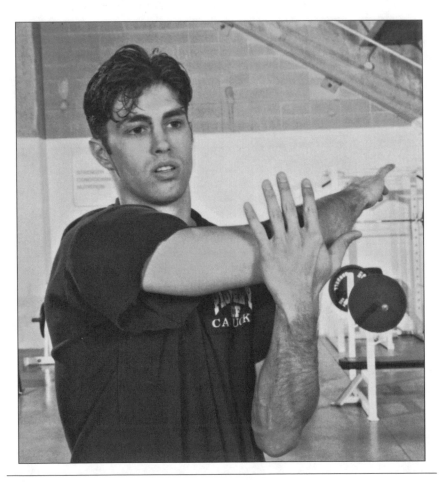

Mike Peca

BICEPS GRIP ON FRAME STRETCH

Focus: Biceps

Procedure: Grasp a frame with your right hand, about lower chest height. Rotate your body around so you're facing away from your hand. Hold for the stretch. Repeat for other arm.

Duration: Hold stretch for 30 seconds.

On-Ice: Use end of plexiglass frame.

OVERHAND GRIP ON FRAME STRETCH

Focus: Upper back

Procedure: Place both hands on a waist high ledge or frame. To accommodate perfect height, set up an Olympic bar across a squat rack. Stand back with your feet flat on the ground and bend over at a 90 degree angle at the waist. To stretch, stay bent over while lowering your hips toward the ground.

Duration: Hold stretch for 30 seconds.

On-Ice: Place gloves atop the boards and lean over toward the boards.

LATERAL SEATED TRUNK STRETCH

Focus: Outside of hip, gluteals, lower back

Procedure: Sit on the floor with your left leg stretched out in front of you. Move your right foot *over* your left leg, placing it flat on the floor above your left knee. Rotate your torso around to the right, placing your right hand behind your body on the floor for support. Your eyes should be looking behind you. Place your left elbow on the outside of your right knee for leverage, although most of the stretch should come from comfortably holding your leg position and rotating your torso. You can push lightly on your knee to assist the stretch. Repeat for other side. (See photo next page)

Duration: Hold stretch for 40 seconds.

On-Ice: Same

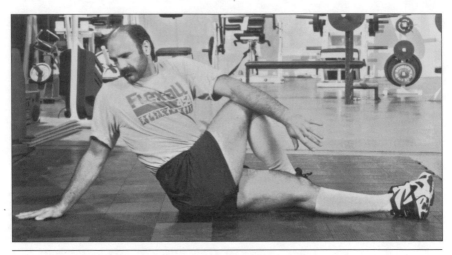

Dave Babych performing the lateral seated trunk stretch.

LYING KNEE TO CHEST STRETCH

Focus: Lower back and gluteals

Procedure: Lying on your back, lack your fingers behind your left knee and pull it up to the chest area. It's important to keep your right leg flat on the ground, even if you cannot move the knee all the way to your chest. Hold the bent leg in a comfortable position. Repeat for other side.

Duration: Hold stretch for 30 seconds.

On-Ice: Same

ABDOMINAL PUSH-UP POSITION STRETCH

Focus: Abdominals

Procedure: Lie face down on the floor in a push-up position, with your hands on the floor at your sides. Push up so your arms are extended and your torso is in the air, but your hips and legs remain on the floor. Hold for the stretch.

Duration: Hold stretch for 40 seconds.

On-Ice: Same

LYING GLUTEAL STRETCH

Focus: Hips and gluteals

Procedure: Lie on your back with your right leg bent, your foot in the air. Take your left foot and place it across your right quadriceps. Grasp both hands around your right hamstring and pull in toward your chin. Repeat other side.

Duration: Hold stretch for 30 seconds.

On-Ice: Same

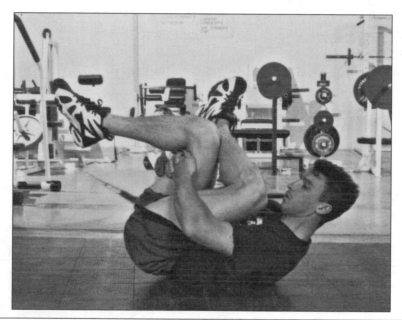

Geoff Courtnall

LYING FORWARD LEAN GLUTEAL STRETCH

Focus: Gluteals, hips

Procedure: Lie on your left side with your left leg bent and your right leg straight. Support your torso with your elbows and your forearms. Keeping your left leg in position, rotate your right leg until it faces the ground, and rotate your torso until your chest faces the ground. Hold for the stretch. Repeat for other side.

Duration: Hold stretch for 30 seconds.

On-Ice: Same

SEATED HAMSTRING STRETCH

Focus: Hamstrings

Procedure: Sit on a bench with your left leg stretched straight out, your foot hanging over the edge. Place your right foot on the floor beside the bench. Move into the stretch by moving your chest straight ahead a few inches. Keep your head up and your torso straight—do not roll your torso just to stretch farther. Hold stretch in a comfortable position. Repeat for opposite leg.

Duration: Hold stretch for 45 seconds.

On-Ice: Stand with your leg up in front of your body, supported by placing your foot atop boards. Lean into the stretch.

STANDING QUADRICEPS/HIP FLEXOR STRETCH

Focus: Quadriceps, hip flexors

Procedure: Move your right foot behind you and atop an object that is waist high or less, supporting your weight with your left foot. Drop your hips straight down toward the floor to stretch the quadriceps. To include more of the hip flexors, move your left foot forward 12 inches, and drop your hips to the floor on an angle toward your support foot. Repeat the stretch with your left foot supported behind your body.

Duration: Hold stretch for 30 seconds.

On-Ice: Place your foot atop boards.

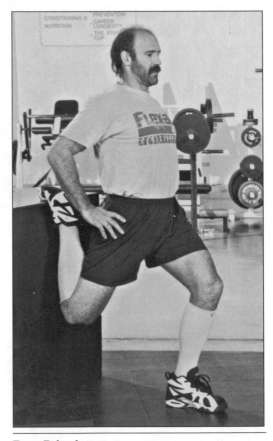

Dave Babych

SEATED GROIN STRETCH

Focus: Groin

Procedure: Sit on the ground with your feet together in front of you, close to your body. Grasp your ankles and place your elbows inside your knees. To stretch, lean forward. To increase the stretch, position your feet closer to your body and increase the forward lean. Do *not* push your elbows into the knees—the groin region must be relaxed to stretch. Your elbows are placed on your knees for posture positioning only, not to apply pressure.

Duration: Hold stretch for 45 seconds.

On-Ice: Kneel on the ice, spread your knees while lowering your hips to the ice and leaning forward with your hands on the ice in front of your body for support.

KNEELING LEG STRETCH

Focus: Quadriceps, ankles, shins

Procedure: Sit in a kneeling position, with your buttocks on your ankles. For an easy stretch, keep your hands on the floor in front of your knees, with your weight forward. To increase the stretch in all three areas, sit more upright, with your hands on the floor at your side. To further progress the stretch, place your hands on the floor behind your ankles, with your weight shifted backward.

Duration: Hold stretch for 30 seconds.

On-Ice: Kneel on the ice with your buttocks on your ankles, sitting upright or leaning back slightly.

STANDING CALF STRETCH

Focus: Calves

Procedure: Stand facing a wall. Place your hands on the wall and one foot on the floor near the wall. Move your opposite foot behind you, placing the toe down and slowly lowering the heel to the floor. Keep your body upright and hold for a stretch. To slightly increase the degree of the stretch, shift your hips forward. The farther your rear foot is from the wall, the greater the stretch, so to reduce the degree of the stretch, place your toe closer to the wall. For a greater stretch, place your toe farther away from the wall.

Duration: Hold stretch for 30 seconds.

DYNAMIC FLEXIBILITY EXERCISES

SNATCH SQUATS

Focus: Quadriceps, hamstrings, groin, gluteals, low back, shoulders

Procedure: Using a wide overhand grip, hold your hockey stick behind and above your head with straight arms. The position of the hockey stick should place a stretch on your shoulders. Using a wide stance, *slowly* lower into a squat position, hold, and return to an upright position.

Duration: Repeat 5 to 10 times.

On-Ice: Same

KNEELING LOWER BODY STRETCH

Focus: Hip flexor, groin, quadriceps, hamstrings

Procedure: Place your right knee on the ground with your left foot flat on the ground out in front of your body. Start with a straight trunk. Lean forward and drop your hips toward the left foot. Hold for the stretch. Repeat with your left foot back and right foot forward. For an increased stretch, place your hands on the floor even with your front foot, one on each side of the foot, and lower your hips farther to the ground. You can also extend your back foot so the top of your foot (shoelace) is in contact with the floor.

Duration: Hold stretch for 40 seconds.

On-Ice: Same

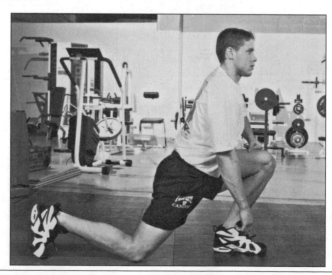

Pavel Bure

HIGH LEG SWINGS

Focus: Hip flexors, extensors, adductors, abductors, lower abdominals

Procedure: Standing upright and balanced on one foot, *slowly* swing your opposite leg forward and back in a smooth arc. Next, swing the leg away from the midline of your body and then bring it back right across in front of your body. You can help balance with one hand on a box or against the wall.

Duration: Perform 10 leg swings each way.

On-Ice: Forward and back leg swings are completed while gliding down ice balanced on one leg. Side-to-side leg swings are better performed using one hand on boards for support.

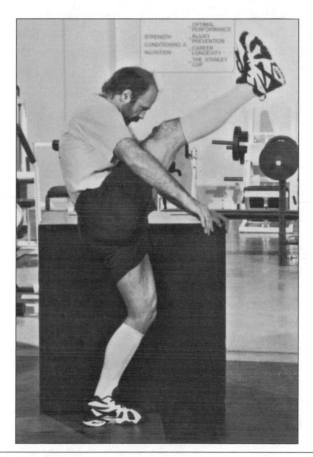

Dave Babych

OUTWARD ROTATIONS

Focus: Hip flexors, abductors, outward rotators

Procedure: Standing on a single leg, bring one knee up to your chest, then outwardly rotate your hips so that your leg moves to the side of your body. Your knee should now be parallel to your shoulder.

Duration: Perform 10 times for each leg.

On-Ice: Complete while gliding down ice balanced on one leg.

TRUNK ROTATION

Focus: Lower back, abdominals, shoulders, chest

Procedure: Holding your stick behind your upper back, slowly and smoothly rotate left and right. Once this has been completed, hold your stick behind your back while leaning forward at the hips. Again, slowly and smoothly rotate.

Duration: Perform stretch for 20 seconds each way.

On-Ice: Complete both ways while gliding around ice balanced evenly on two skates.

ARM SWINGS

Focus: Shoulders

Procedure: Stand upright with your knees slightly bent. Keep one arm relaxed at your side; with the opposite arm, complete forward circles. Keep your arm fairly straight and close to your body as it circles. Your arm and hand should be very close to your head as it circles up top. Use a slow and smooth motion, in a big arc. Repeat backward. Repeat with your other arm.

Duration: Perform 10 circles each way with each arm.

On-Ice: Complete on-ice while gliding. You can hold your stick in your relaxed arm, or try it in the active arm for light loading.

WIDE STICKHANDLING

Focus: Arms, abdominals, low back

Procedure: In a stationary position, with your knees slightly bent, hold a stick. With or without a puck or ball, take the stick through an exaggerated stickhandling pattern. Move through wide loops in a slow and smooth motion. You can also hold your stick upside down and use a 5- or 10-pound Olympic weight for some light loading, placing the end of the stick in the middle of the weight.

Duration: 30 seconds

On-Ice: Complete while gliding around ice. Then try with slow strides, moving from one leg to the next, but make sure you use an exaggerated, wide loop with the stick. Use a puck to complete wide and slow stickhandling.

CHAPTER 3

AEROBIC AND ANAEROBIC TRAINING

Your body has different energy systems that work together to fuel hockey performance. The aerobic system provides energy for low- and moderate-intensity exercise and helps the body recover from fatigue. The anaerobic systems produce energy very quickly to meet the demands of intense action, such as a slapshot, sprinting on a breakaway, or stop-and-starts while penalty killing.

In this chapter, I'll explain how your body's energy systems contribute to hockey performance and how you can best prepare these systems to meet the demands of an intense hockey game.

AEROBIC ENERGY

Aerobic power refers to energy produced by the aerobic energy system (also known as the oxygen system). Its level is determined by measuring the rate at which the body can breathe in oxygen to the lungs, transfer oxygen from the lungs to the heart, deliver the oxygen through the blood to the working muscles, extract the oxygen from the blood to the muscles, and use the oxygen in the muscles for energy production. Aerobic power is expressed as $\dot{V}O_2$max, the maximum volume of oxygen that can be taken up and used by the body (ml/kg–min).

The aerobic energy system supplies energy for low-intensity exercise for a long duration. A one-hour bike ride at a comfortable pace, for example, would be fueled mainly by the aerobic system. The aerobic system is a

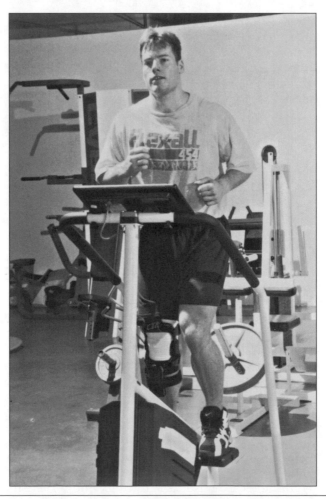

Martin Gelinas getting an aerobic workout on a stair-climbing machine.

system of supply and recovery: It supplies energy for submaximal efforts and helps players recover after very intense action. A strong aerobic base allows a player to work longer and at a higher intensity by postponing fatigue and allowing a speedy recovery. During conditioning work, an aerobic base helps athletes recover between sets and between workouts.

Hockey is characterized by repeated bouts of high-intensity action interspersed with periods of moderate activity and active rest (during play stoppages). The aerobic energy system supplies a small portion of the energy needed during intense efforts and most of the energy needed during moderate activity, and it is critical for efficient recovery between play stoppages and during time on the bench. You rely on the aerobic system when you come off the ice from your last shift and sit on the bench, out of breath, breathing very hard, and trying to take in more oxygen. The more ice time a player has—the longer the shifts and the shorter the bench time—the more important the aerobic system is for recovery.

General aerobic fitness is important in hockey because the body uses both specific and nonspecific muscle fibers to recover between shifts. Skating mainly relies on fast-twitch muscle fibers, but nonspecific slow-twitch muscle fibers also take up lactic acid and contribute to recovery. So building aerobic fitness through exercises like running or stair-climbing that use muscles nonspecific to ice hockey will still benefit the hockey player during a game.

A high $\dot{V}O_2$ max will also help players recover more quickly between games. In addition, postgame aerobic exercise will accelerate the recovery process. An easy 15- to 20-minute bike ride following intense games or practices will help remove lactic acid from your legs. Light exercise postgame or postpractice speeds leg recovery. Likewise, light skating between play stoppages or between drills also helps the legs recover.

"Aerobic fitness helps both your game performance and your recovery," says Paul Coffey. "I include aerobic activity in my off-season conditioning program by riding a stationary bike or cycling to and from the golf course on my mountain bike. Plus, I swim and rollerblade. In-season, I bike, bike, bike. After a hard game, it's good for getting the lactic acid out of your legs, for recovery. Or if I didn't have a good game, or the game didn't really get my heart pumping with a real burn in my legs, then I'll ride the bike after the game, for fitness."

AEROBIC CONDITIONING

There are two ways to improve aerobic conditioning: through sub-maximal continuous exercise and through high-intensity, intermittent exercise. Submaximal continuous exercise at 75 to 85 percent of

Paul Coffey

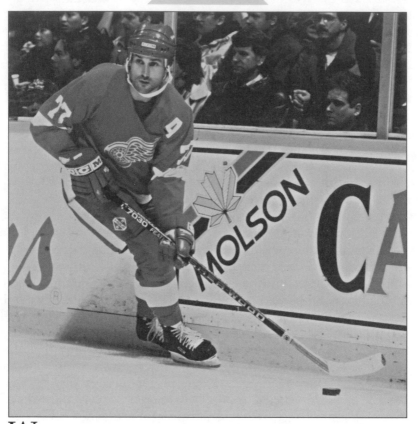

Well recognized as one of the best skaters in hockey, Paul Coffey's legs have supported him through 16 NHL seasons. He has been a standout through more than 1,200 NHL games, scoring over 1,500 points while tallying up many individual accomplishments: 13 All-Star Games, three Norris Trophies as the NHL's best defenseman, and the NHL's all-time leading scorer for defensemen, topping the list for goals, assists, and points.

"I know personally, I'm in better shape now than I was 16 years ago," Coffey says. "When I broke into the league 16 years ago, we had a training camp that was several weeks long. At that time you were able to come to camp overweight and out of shape. Now, if you don't report to camp in great shape, you're going to be lost. The demands on the athlete in today's game are incredibly high." Conditioning has progressed to a year-round, structured commitment. "Sixteen years ago, hockey was an 8-month job for me, so to speak, says Coffey. "Now it is 11$\frac{1}{2}$ months. You can usually afford the luxury of having a couple of weeks off at the end of the season. But the key to staying in shape is not getting out of shape. Everyone who has been out of shape knows what a grind it is to get back into shape."

Coffey's individual abilities and achievements cumulated in the ultimate team accomplishment. He won three Stanley Cup Championships with the Edmonton Oilers in the mid-1980s and a fourth in 1991, quarterbacking the Pittsburgh Penguins to hockey's supremacy. He now tops all defensemen, scoring the most career playoff points of any defenseman. The world's best athletes have one thing in common: They continually search for ways to improve. With each new level they reach, every success they achieve, they remain open to ideas on how to keep improving. "It's important to keep trying to consistently improve," Coffey says. Athletes should always be in a stage of improvement, and be willingly trying to get better. "I think I'm still there. I *know* I'm still there," confirms Coffey. "Of course I'm finding easier ways to do things on the ice, and better ways to play the game, but your conditioning is so important. You shouldn't lock yourself out from anything—there's always room to improve.

"I was fortunate my first year, 1981, when I went to the Canada Cup. At that time they had a bunch of older guys there. I was 19 years old, and the team had players like Larry Robinson and Dennis Potvin. Larry was 30 years old at the time. To me, at 19, 30 was just *old*. I wondered how he was still playing the game. I kind of idolized Larry and had a lot of respect for him, so I hung around with him a bit. I remember saying to him, 'What's your key to still being able to play at this level?' What he told me really stuck in my mind. Larry said, 'If you take care of your body, your body will take care of you. And that's something you can't start when you're 30 years old. You have to start doing it early in your career.' So I started doing that—conditioning, nutrition, hard work—and it has really helped me."

maximum heart rate for 30 to 60 minutes will improve the heart's ability to deliver oxygen to the muscles for energy and will allow the body to recover more quickly from intense efforts. Intermittent aerobic conditioning using a series of 2 to 3 minutes of higher intensity exercise (five beats below maximum heart rate at the end of each interval) interspersed with 2 to 3 minutes of relief (active rest) phases, builds the aerobic supply system and increases the muscles' ability to extract oxygen from the blood.

Athletes should first use long-duration continuous aerobic exercise to build up a base of fitness, then progress to intermittent aerobic conditioning. As previously mentioned, since continuous aerobic exercise develops your lungs' and heart's capabilities, aerobic exercise of any sort will benefit athletes, but because intermittent aerobic conditioning additionally stimulates changes in the working muscles, it is important to select intermittent exercise that is more specific to the skating muscles.

Both continuous and intermittent exercises help raise the lactate threshold of muscles (the point where lactic acid accumulation exceeds its utilization and removal). Lactic acid build-up ultimately limits on-ice activity because it indirectly interferes with working muscles and leads to fatigue.

By raising their lactate threshold, athletes can perform at higher intensities aerobically without having to anaerobically meet energy demands, thereby delaying lactic acid accumulation (see figure 3.1) and preserving glycogen stores needed for energy production. Improved aerobic fitness also increases the efficiency of the body's cooling system and can lead to lower body fat—very important for efficient movement on the ice.

Table 3.1 gives exercise guidelines for designing an aerobic conditioning program. Hockey players should seek to build the aerobic base in the off-season to prepare for the more intense demands of preseason conditioning. Because in-season on-ice activity often does not build up aerobic power, and because hockey schedules do not leave enough time to fit in long off-ice aerobic workouts, aerobic fitness is best developed through off-ice endurance training in the off-season. During the season, aerobic conditioning needs to be tailored according to the intensity and frequency of games.

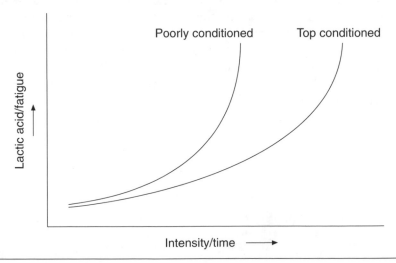

Figure 3.1 The relationship between level of conditioning and fatigue. Better conditioned players can compete at a higher intensity with less lactic acid accumulation and compete longer with fatiguing.

Table 3.1   Aerobic Conditioning Variables

Type	Continuous	Intermittent
Intensity	75 to 85% maximum heart rate	5 beats below maximum heart rate
Work time	30 to 60 minutes	2½ minutes
Work-to-rest ratio	N/A	1:1
Reps and sets	N/A	6 to 10
Frequency	4 to 5 times per week	3 times per week

Aerobic conditioning is often the day's first phase of exercise, designed to leave the athlete well warmed up for what comes next. Or it is left until the end of the workout to facilitate recovery. I recommend using a variety of sports during conditioning rather than structured aerobic exercises, especially for younger athletes. I've seen some hockey players who have played exclusively hockey from an early age—they not only face burnout and being turned off the sport, but also lack an overall athletic base. Their limitations during exercises that require unique balance and coordination skills is often apparent.

OFF-ICE AEROBIC EXERCISES

Off-ice aerobic exercises can include road cycling, stationary cycling, stair-climbing, and running. During runs, I like to include backward and sideways running, as well as directional changes and footwork. Hiking mountain trails is a great aerobic conditioner—the irregular terrain is good for developing single-leg balance, coordination, and stabilizer muscles. Changing terrain also helps build strength around the hips, knees, and ankles, whereas hiking inclines builds leg power.

In-line skating is good for aerobic conditioning, but the exact skating technique differs from hockey skating, so if used too frequently you'll end up practicing and learning incorrect ice skating technique. After a full summer of daily in-line skating, players discover at training camp that their on-ice skating technique is off. They feel like they are on their toes too much and have difficulty stopping and making sharp pivots. In-line skating for a long duration causes fatigue, which can result in a complete breakdown in technique. For these reasons, I use in-line skating for intermittent aerobic intervals no more than a couple of times per week, and I mix them with other exercise modes.

Circuit training, another valuable aerobic conditioner, involves alternating a set of weight training—light weight and high reps—with aerobic exercise. For example, the athlete may lift a weight for 45 seconds and then ride a stationary bike or perform step-ups on a box for 45 seconds. This continues back and forth from strength exercise to aerobic exercise throughout the session.

The athlete can progress through a variety of weight training exercises to work all the major muscle groups. This spreads the weight training around so that fatigue does not limit the duration of this exercise routine. The combination of aerobic exercise interspersed with light weight training is a very effective conditioner.

ON-ICE AEROBIC EXERCISES

FIGURE-8 AEROBIC SKATE

Purpose: To build aerobic fitness and oxygen extraction capabilities of skating muscles.

Procedure:

1. The posts of the net are moved even with the face-off circle hashmarks so that the distance from net to net is 160 feet.

2. Skate continuously around each net and through the center in an elongated figure-8.

3. Complete as many laps as possible in 12 minutes, skate for a set duration, or complete aerobic intervals, skating for $2^1/_2$ minutes then resting while teammates complete an interval, repeating several times.

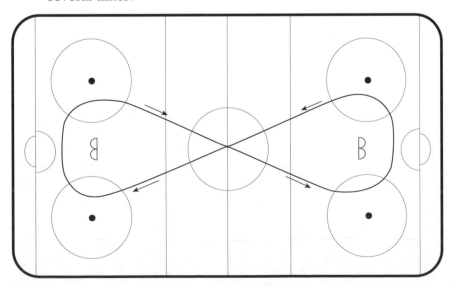

AEROBIC CIRCLE DRILL

Purpose: To develop aerobic fitness and oxygen extraction capabilities of skating muscles.

Procedure:

1. Start at the goal line in the corner and skate around circle 1.
2. Skate down the boards and around circle 2.
3. Skate diagonally across ice and around circle 3.
4. Skate down boards and around circle 4.
5. Skate diagonally back to the starting position.
6. Continue drill for two minutes. Rest for two minutes. Complete a total of six reps. For two of the reps, skate backward through the course.

Start

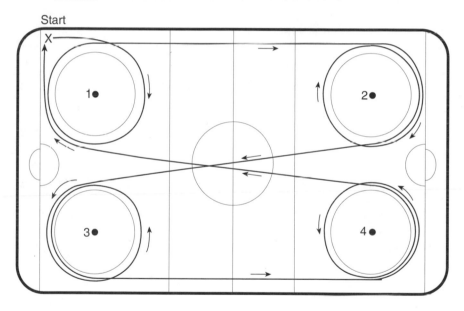

ANAEROBIC ENERGY SYSTEMS

The anaerobic energy systems provide the major source of energy during a hockey game. Since hockey is a stop-and-start sport involving repetitive sprinting situations, athletes must be able to react to a situation and explode into action by exerting maximum effort over short distances. Such movements place demands on the anaerobic systems.

The first anaerobic energy system, the *ATP-PC system,* provides the most immediate form of energy. It is used for bursts of maximum-intensity exercise for up to 10 seconds—explosive starts, bodychecks, and shooting would fall into this category. After 10 seconds of intense action, continuation at an intense level depends on the second anaerobic method of energy supply—the *lactic acid system*. Also referred to as *anaerobic glycolysis*, this system draws upon your muscle glycogen or blood glucose stores (carbohydrates) for energy.

Anaerobic glycolysis provides an important energy supply for hockey shifts. Its energy production has an upper limit of 120 seconds, depending on intensity, but peaks at 30 to 45 seconds. This is why the typical hockey shift averages 45 seconds in duration. Intense shifts that last much longer will be characterized by fatigue, submaximal efforts, and deteriorating skill execution.

Fatigue is related to a build-up of lactic acid—a by-product of the anaerobic glycolysis energy system—that accumulates in the muscles and the blood. Stopping and starting, sprinting, fighting through checks, and battling one-on-one for the puck require intense efforts that produce lactic acid in both the upper and lower body. With lactic acid accumulation, your muscles take longer to contract and suffer a decreased rate of relaxation between contractions, which leads to slower movement and the stiffness or burning you feel in your legs at the end of a shift. Because lactic acid indirectly hinders your muscles' ability to move, skill and technique are adversely affected by its build-up.

During a game, the two anaerobic energy systems and the aerobic energy system are active for each and every shift. If you need a high rate of energy supply for explosive acceleration or a quick shot from the point, the ATP-PC system is drawn upon. Longer duration intense action uses anaerobic glycolysis. Submaximal efforts and between shift recovery are fueled by the aerobic system (see figure 3.2). While each of the three systems has its specialty, at no time does any one energy system provide the entire supply of energy needed for a movement. Rather, the three energy systems are drawn upon at the same time, and the extent

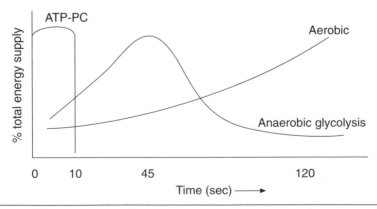

Figure 3.2   Relative contribution of the three energy systems over time.

to which each responds depends on the intensity and duration of the activity, the player's fitness level and skating efficiency, and the game situation. Killing a penalty, forechecking, and bodychecking all change the relative contribution of the three energy systems. Likewise, there are easy shifts and intense shifts.

Anaerobic Conditioning

Poorly conditioned legs fatigue early. When fatigued, players cannot generate much stride power. They tend to straighten their legs and have little "jump" in their stride. When players alter their skating technique to compensate in an effort to get some stride power, flawed technique results. Fatigued players with straightened legs tend to slow down, stumble, and are more easily knocked down by their opponents. To handle sharp pivots, high-speed crossovers, explosive acceleration, and crushing blows, it's important for players to maintain a deep knee-bend, with hips low and their knee over the front foot. By improving anaerobic conditioning, players can achieve this for longer periods.

Anaerobic conditioning raises the lactate threshold, which allows players to compete at a higher intensity before the accumulation of lactic acid exceeds its removal. The energy production system becomes more efficient, as less lactic acid is produced at a given work intensity. Intense anaerobic conditioning also promotes lactic acid toleration, so that once your legs are fatigued and lactic acid builds up, you are accustomed to the feeling. Training develops the mental strength needed to keep playing for a few more seconds. This could be critical when stuck in your end for a long time killing a penalty, or at the end of a shift when you block a shot at the point and suddenly have a breakaway opportunity.

To be properly prepared for the extreme demands of hockey, players need to condition at a higher intensity than they will face during a game. Conditioning needs to be periodized throughout a season, during which there will be recovery days and light practices, but also times of super-intense workouts. "It is better to do a 20-minute workout *all-out* than 40 minutes at half-speed," stresses George Nevole, head strength and conditioning coach at Cornell University. Today's practices feature more flow drills than ever before. "You need flow for today's game," says Dave Babych. "But you still need short sprints and stop-and-starts to prepare your legs for killing penalties and exploding into action."

Sprint Intervals

To develop anaerobic energy systems, players should use *sprint intervals*. These involve a full-out, high-intensity, high-speed interval

Pat Quinn, President and General Manager
of the Vancouver Canucks

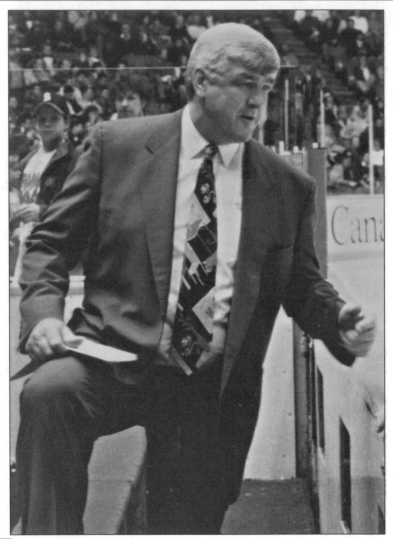

Pat Quinn played nine seasons in the NHL as a hard-hitting defenseman. As a player throughout the 1970s, Quinn experienced first hand the change from a game that placed no emphasis on physical preparation and no practice structure to one that began to implement practice drills and then later included on-ice and off-ice conditioning. He was on the leading edge for emphasizing conditioning while combining physical development with the coaching process. "When I played, teams didn't pay any attention to preparation. When I first started, practices just involved warming up the goaltenders, then scrimmaging. Somehow I met some runners who were interested in testing and training. They tested my aerobic fitness, and this was the first time I started to pay attention to my preparation. I played one more year, then I got into coaching and carried the interest in fitness into my coaching. When I started coaching in Philadelphia, I still hadn't been involved in strength training. They had some basic equipment set up, and I commissioned some studies on sport conditioning and implemented preseason testing. When I started coaching in LA they were not a training team, so I hired an exercise physiologist to consult us on conditioning. We experimented with practice times, travel schedules, practice plans, and all kinds of things directed toward trying to get better performance results. Then I came to Vancouver, who already had coaches who were interested in conditioning. Conditioning is important to success at all levels, both individually and for the team. Without question, conditioning is a key factor in our team's success."

Quinn first won the NHL Coach of the Year Award with the Philadelphia Flyers, where he coached from 1978 to 1982. After earning a law degree, he returned to coaching with Los Angeles, from 1984 to 1987, also coaching Team Canada in 1986. With the Vancouver Canucks, Quinn was named the *Hockey News* Executive of the Year in 1992 while winning the NHL Coach of the Year award the same season. He led Vancouver to the Stanley Cup Finals in 1994.

"On the West Coast, we have fewer practice days, so to work enough on team systems, we have to do some of our conditioning off-ice. It's imperative that minor hockey coaches adopt a similar approach. If we only have two good practices one week, most of the ice time is needed for the tactical and technical approach to coaching, as opposed to the conditioning part of coaching. So to fit in teaching and coaching team systems and individual skills, conditioning must be supplemented off the ice. Time is needed for players to practice individual skills—passing, skating, stickhandling. But the conditioning that is needed to develop hockey skills has to be done sometime, so coaches need to take their athletes through dry-land practices. Developing a skill takes time and requires repetition and discipline. Those are things that are often done through a dry-land session if you don't have the time to do everything on the ice. Conditioning can start at a young age; in fact, young players *must* have specific muscle development or else they'll never skate properly, because they'll learn it imperfectly."

While young players need good coaching for their physical development and skill learning, Quinn identifies a problem with the emphasis on only hockey. "One thing I don't like about our game today is that one sport takes too much time from the kids. If they're hockey players when they're seven, it's a 12-month job now, with summer camps and a heavy game schedule. This works against overall development of skill and athletic ability. I'd much rather see kids play as many team sports as they can."

followed by a rest or active relief interval. For anaerobic glycolysis, use 45-second work intervals, which are specific to the length of a hockey shift and correlate with anaerobic glycolysis' peak energy production. During initial anaerobic conditioning, you may use 30-second work intervals as a break-in period.

The early stages of anaerobic interval training use a work-to-rest ratio of 1:5 or 1:4, which is an optimal ratio for developing anaerobically. (A 1:1 work-to-rest ratio involves sprinting all-out for 45 seconds, active recovery for 45 seconds, then sprinting full-out again for 45 seconds, and so on.) It is also appropriate for initial workouts, providing adequate recovery time between each sprint. With subsequent anaerobic workouts, I decrease the relief period to close in on the actual game situation. Specific to hockey, a forward may have a 1:3 or 1:2 work-to-rest ratio, while some defensemen have a 1:1 work-to-rest ratio.

Players should complete six to ten of these sprint interval repetitions. How quickly players progress to shorter work-relief ratios will depend on their abilities to sustain full-out efforts for the 45-second work phase.

The best way to recover from intense anaerobic sprints is with active recovery, but the sport of hockey forces players to recover sitting on a crowded bench with their legs stationary and cramped in a tight space. Optimal recommendations include more room for the players to stretch their legs, or room for a type of bike pedal set-up in front of the bench that would allow the players to lightly move their legs, or a small strip of ice behind the bench on which players can recover between shifts. To deal with the current design of rinks, have players go right to the bench and sit down for their rest interval during some anaerobic drills.

It's important to structure some sprint drills to specifically develop the ATP-PC system. Speed and quickness drills incorporate shorter intervals and longer rest periods, precisely what is needed to optimally develop the ATP-PC system. Anaerobic glycolysis drills result in enough muscle fatigue and leg discomfort that they force players to adhere to a between-sprint rest period—players need and want to rest. But ATP-PC sprint intervals require greater coach control. See table 3.2 for a comparison of the ATP-PC system and anaerobic glycolysis.

To develop the ATP-PC system, athletes must work under full-out, sprint conditions and then allow enough time for the energy supply to replenish itself to fuel the next sprint repetition. Additionally, sprints must be kept short (2 to 10 seconds) to condition this system. If sprint intervals are not done full-out, if they are too long, or if rest intervals are too short, you will *not* build the ATP-PC system, build speed, or develop quickness and agility—you will actually learn to be slow.

To achieve these conditioning gains, rest intervals are absolutely critical. Players are so used to being pushed harder and harder—to full fatigue—that they're not satisfied with very short sprints followed by long rest periods. If they only sprint for 5 seconds, not anywhere close to fatiguing, they don't understand why they should take a 30-second rest, especially since coaches always push them in the opposite direction.

There are appropriate times for overloading athletes, for pushing them past their physical endurance limits, but ATP-PC, speed, and quickness and agility training is *quality* training, not quantity. For time efficiency, or to make coaches and players more comfortable with the rest periods, use the rest times for instruction or for practicing well-learned skills under a partially fatigued (game-like) condition.

Table 3.2 Anaerobic Conditioning Variables

	ATP-PC	Anaerobic glycolysis
Type	Sprint intervals	Sprint intervals
Intensity	Full-out	Full-out
Work time	2 to 10 seconds	30 to 45 seconds
Work-to-rest	1:5 W:R	Start 1:5 or 1:4 W:R Progress to 1:1 W:R
Reps and sets	Start 10 reps, 1 set Progress to 10 reps, 2 sets	Start 6 reps, 1 set Progress to 10 reps, 1 set
Rest between sets	3 minutes rest	N/A
Frequency	2 to 3 times per week	2 to 3 times per week

OFF-ICE ANAEROBIC EXERCISES

ATP-PC	Anaerobic Glycolysis
Stair sprinting	Slideboard (retain deep knee position)
Skipping	Stationary bike sprints
Quickness and agility drills (see chapter 5)	In-line skating
Speed drills (see chapter 6)	400-yard running sprints
Plyometrics (see chapter 5)	Hill running/cycling
Explosive strength training (see chapter 4)	

ON-ICE ANAEROBIC EXERCISES

The following drills incorporate sprint intervals with rest periods—ideal for developing the energy systems. For more anaerobic energy building drills, see the on-ice activities in chapters 5 and 6.

ATP-PC SPRINT START RELAYS

Purpose: To improve the ATP-PC energy system and explosive starting abilities.

Procedure:

1. In this diagram, a team of 20 players is working off of four face-off circles, using all players, for 5-yard sprint relays.

2. On the whistle, the first player (1, 6, 11, 16) in each group sprints toward his teammate.

3. The second player (2, 7, 12, 17) maintains a stationary ready stance until the first player touches glove to glove.

4. The second player sprints to the next one in line.

5. Five players per group gives a 1:4 work-to-rest ratio.

6. Each player completes three reps, racing against the other groups.

7. Rest before repeating the team sprint relay again.

8. Try using three distances: 20 yards (blue to blue), 10 yards (red to blue), and 5 yards (face-off dot to edge of circle).

Tips:

- Use four different stationary starts—forward, backward, and sideways (left and right start).

- Emphasize the first two strides for starting explosion and stride frequency.

- Watch for glove contact and false starts (too soon, not in position).

- Players should not rise up too soon, staying low for a powerful stride.

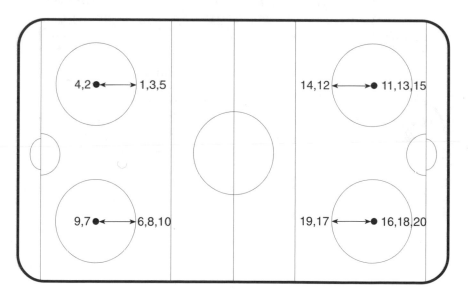

PAIR RACE DRILL

Purpose: To develop the anaerobic glycolysis system and practice performing skills under a partially fatigued condition.

Procedure:

1. Two players (A and B) start together, on the whistle, at the face-off dot (a second pair from the other line of players—C and D—start at the same time from diagonally opposite corner).

2. Stop at center red, back to the blue, and on down the ice.

3. Once players cross the center red line, skaters get a pass from the last two players in line at the boards.

4. The lead skater—the first one to cross the center red line (in this case player A)—shoots from top of slot. Trailing skater has to attack right to net for a deke, skating straight down the boards and moving across the low slot.

5. After shooting, players immediately turn up ice and complete the same pattern down the opposite side. This places emphasis on the first sprint—trailing skater ends up with longer skate down both sides of ice.

6. Next two pairs start at the face-off dot on the coach's whistle.

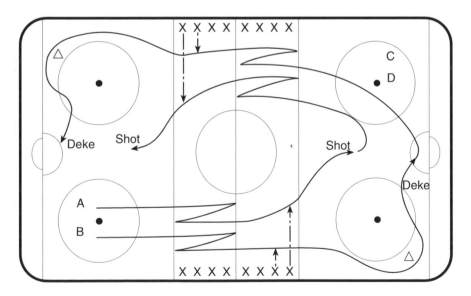

ANAEROBIC LINE DRILL

Purpose: To develop the anaerobic glycolysis system and lactic acid toleration.

Procedure:

1. Split the team into thirds.
2. Line up the first one-third of the team across the goal red line.
3. Players stop and start, sprinting through drill as quickly as possible.
4. On whistle, sprint to the blue line (1) and back (2).
5. Immediately sprint from the goal red line to the center red line (3), and back to the start (4).
6. Next, sprint down to the far blue line (5) and back to the goal red line (6).
7. To finish, skate right down to the far red goal line (7) and back to the start (8).
8. Players rest for two turns, while the other two-thirds of the team completes, for a 1:2 work-to-rest ratio.
9. Repeat three to six times.

Tips:

- Players should stop facing the same side of the ice each time, to get equal practice stopping and starting left and right.
- For one set of the line drill, have players skate forward down ice to line and backward to return to start.
- Players can pivot at each line for a modified line drill.

Start

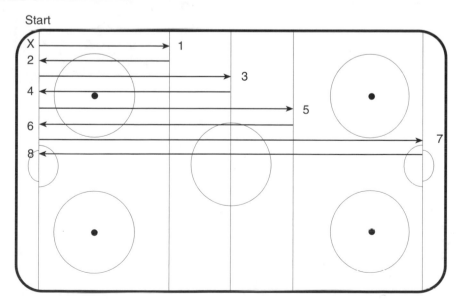

DOT-TO-DOT DRILL

Purpose: To increase lactic acid toleration and mental toughness and develop the anaerobic glycolysis system.

Procedure:

1. Start on first face-off dot.

2. Sprint to second face-off dot (arrow 1), full stop, sprint back to original dot (arrow 2), full stop, then sprint past second face-off dot right on through to third face-off dot (arrow 3), full stop, sprint back to second dot (arrow 4), and so on, right around ice.

3. Stop and start facing middle of ice, to work both sides equally and to always "face the play."

4. Stay in line with face-off dots—arrows on diagram are spread out for visual clarity only.

Tips:

- A clear coaching cue is to "skate two down and one back."

- Coaches, give verbal encouragement for athletes to persevere and push themselves through last half of the drill.

- Full stop-and-start each dot.

- Stress, even when fatigued and legs are tight, exploding off each dot as fast as possible.

- To modify this drill, pivot around each dot.

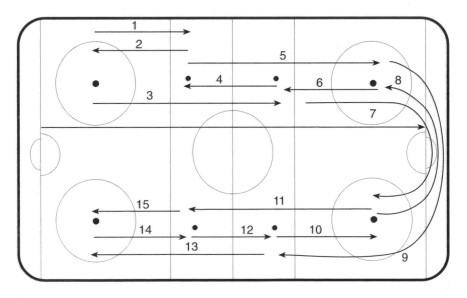

TWO-LAP PACED DRILL

Purpose: To develop anaerobic glycolysis system.

Procedure:

1. Move nets up to hashmarks.
2. Players will skate two laps and then rest.
3. Assuming 20 players on a team, line up 10 on each side of the ice in the neutral zone.
4. The first two players in line pair up and are ready at the center red line.
5. On whistle, the first pair from each side sprints two laps.
6. Once first pair completes one lap, second pair in line joins in and pushes the first pair to maintain their speed through the second lap. The goal for the skaters in the first pair is to not get passed by the second pair.
7. Third pair gets ready to join in on the second pairs' second lap.
8. The fourth pair joins in on the third pairs' second lap.
9. Continue cycling through pairs.

Tips:

- This gives a 1:1.5 work-to-rest ratio. For longer or shorter rest periods, group players accordingly. Players can go one at a time or in threes.
- Manipulate the number of players per group according to the number of players on your team and the work-to-rest ratio you want.
- You can also work groups out of just one line, to achieve the desired work-to-rest ratio.

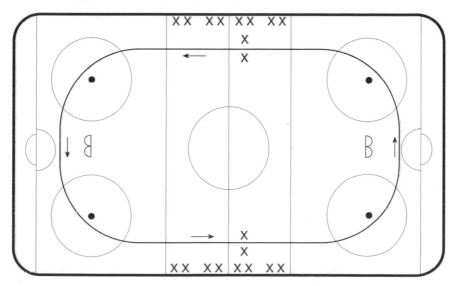

POSITION/SHIFT-SPECIFIC DRILL

Purpose: To develop anaerobic glycolysis system with a sport-specific recovery set-up.

Procedure:

1. On whistle, the first wave of players hop boards and complete as many laps around the rink as possible in 30 seconds.

2. On second whistle, players move to their position location and complete stop-and-starts through the pattern for 15 seconds.

3. On third whistle, players skate over to bench and sit down, while next wave of players hop boards and begin 30 seconds of laps.

4. Goaltenders skate from their crease around behind the net and back again, alternating sides for full 15 seconds.

5. Defensemen skate from in front of the net to the corner, backward to the front of the net, forward to face-off dot, and backward to front of net for 15 seconds.

6. Forwards forecheck to end boards, skate over to side boards, then sprint to top of slot, continuing for 15 seconds.

Tips:

- Manipulate your line combinations and player groupings to achieve your desired work-to-rest ratio.

- Sound the second whistle at 25 seconds to give players five seconds to move into position.

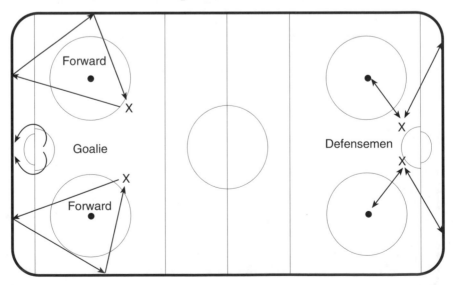

CHAPTER 4

STRENGTH TRAINING

A solid base of strength and lean muscle mass supports a player's physical abilities and technical skills and is a prerequisite to anaerobic conditioning, power, quickness, agility, and speed. Strength assists such skating skills as acceleration, cornering, stopping and starting, pivoting, shooting, and dynamic balance. Increased size and strength are also important for bodychecking and defending opponents.

Both absolute strength and relative strength are important to on-ice performance. Hockey requires absolute strength (total muscular strength), as players must have the mass and power to move others and to withstand contact. Relative strength (strength in relation to body weight) fosters quickness, agility, and speed.

Improved strength and musculature protects players from injury by building strength around the joints—important because the primary cause of musculoskeletal injury is inadequate strength. Physical preparation is vital for a high-speed, high-collision sport like hockey in which explosive movements can injure unprepared muscles. "You have to be very strong and flexible in all parts of your body, through every angle and every movement pattern," says Curt Fraser. "Hockey's a game where you're going to get hit from all sides, and your body must be prepared to handle that." When injuries do occur, they'll be less severe and will mend much quicker if the player has built up a solid base of muscular strength.

Upper-body strength contributes to shooting and puck control, as well as warding off opponents. Strength through the chest, shoulders, arms, and back is used during bodychecking, to clear the slot, or when containing your opponent against the boards.

As in golf, your upper-body movement is an extension of the movement from your legs and torso—thus, overall strength is crucial to

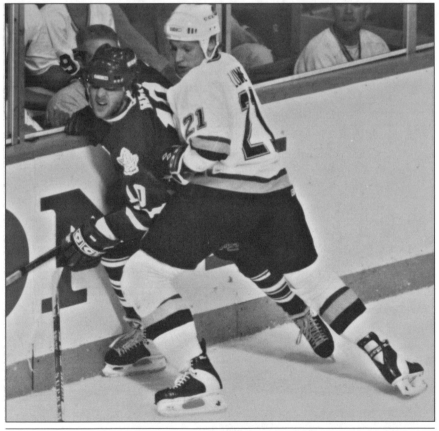

As you can see by the technique Jyrki Lumme uses to contain his man, successful bodychecking requires strength of both the lower and the upper body.

support the upper body. For instance, a bodycheck initiates with the legs and hips and is followed through by the arms. Even while a player is pinning an opponent against the boards with the arm, the torso region is contracted to stabilize the effort, while the legs continue to balance the body and drive toward the opponent.

Leg strength is important to skating strides, acceleration, turning, and stopping. It contributes to first-step leg power for a strong pushoff and anaerobic endurance for repetitive strides. Successful bodychecking also relies on strong legs. Weight shifts upward during a bodycheck, with 75 percent of the power coming from the legs.

Building leg muscle mass lowers the body's center of gravity, assisting dynamic balance and stability, enabling a player to skate through resistance from opponents. For a hockey player, "it is more important to develop mass in the lower body," says Lorne Goldenberg, strength and conditioning coach for the Ottawa Senators. "By lowering the center of gravity, players have the strength to bend their knees more to make tighter turns. A hockey player with a big upper body and no legs will fall over in tight, high-speed turns."

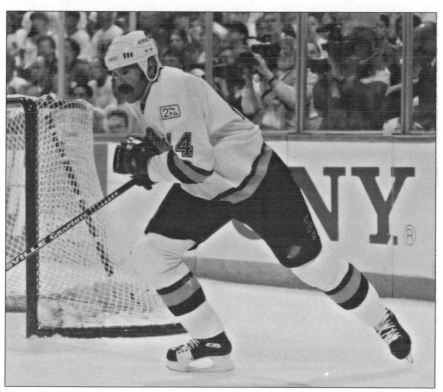

Dave Babych using a long, powerful stride.

The value of lower-body strength is recognized by one of the game's best skaters, Paul Coffey of the Detroit Red Wings. "I think that every part of your body has to be strong, but first and foremost is your skating. In this league, with today's players, you have to be an above average or a great skater to really succeed at the game. I think all that comes from leg strength. If you have strong legs, they'll carry you a long way through your career."

Other muscles are also very important to skating. The torso serves as the body's base, its pillar, from which all movement stems. The torso initiates, assists, and stabilizes movement. Every on-ice action relies on the abdominals, lower back, and hip region. Stronger legs will not improve one aspect of your game without torso strength. Every stride, from the drive phase to the recovery phase, relies on torso strength. Quick turns and directional changes on the ice come from the legs, lower back, abdominals, and hips. All on-ice strength, power, speed, quickness, and agility stem from the torso out to the legs and arms. "I concentrate on building lower-body strength to improve my skating, because if you can't skate, you can't play," says Jyrki Lumme. "Leg and torso strength is the first thing young players should develop. If you can skate well, you can develop all other areas of your game easier."

During shooting and checking, the player rotates at the hips and applies force outside the body's center of gravity. This places incredible demands on the low back and abdominals, which are the first areas that will break down. Inadequate strength in the torso limits explosive skating, agility, shooting, and checking. Poor torso strength leaves a player injured after attempting a single explosive or forceful action, or through overuse from repetitive explosive rotational movements.

"There's a whole different set of injuries than there was 10 years ago," says Steve Larmer of the New York Rangers' 1994 Stanley Cup team. "You're seeing a lot more abdominal strains and a lot more back problems, and I think it's because the players are a lot bigger, they're a lot stronger, and they're much faster. Everybody is so big and so strong, you really have to strain to fight through a check or to hit somebody."

Strength training exercises that involve a full range of motion will actually improve flexibility, and enhanced strength through this entire range of motion will help players control on-ice movements, complementing fluid and agile actions.

DEVELOPING A STRENGTH TRAINING PROGRAM

Along with the basic conditioning principles presented in chapter 1, use the following strength-specific guidelines when developing a strength

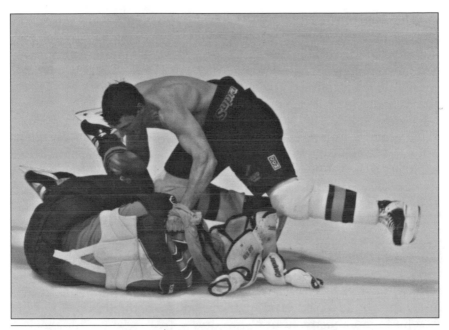

Torso strength, dynamic balance, single-leg strength, and upper-body strength all help Gino Odjick win physical confrontations—this time against the St. Louis Blues.

training program. Remember that young athletes and players with little conditioning experience should spend time using very light loads and concentrating on technique. They need time to develop a base of strength while working on correct form and balance. Technique is important for exercise safety and strength results.

Intensity

Weight training is organized by sets and repetitions (reps). A *rep* is one complete range of motion with a weight for a particular exercise. A group of reps comprise a *set*—the number of reps performed without resting.

The more intense your workout, the greater the strength development. The load for a given exercise is best determined by the number of repetitions, the rest time between sets, and the speed of movement. In general, hockey players should work within 6 to 15 repetitions. For a 10-rep set, you estimate a weight that will cause fatigue on the tenth rep. By the second set, after a minor adjustment in the weight, you should fatigue at exactly 10 reps. No other system is more accurate than this—it is a truly individualized loading system and helps athletes learn what their muscles can handle and how they respond.

Rest time between sets affects the amount of weight you can lift, as well as the muscular strength/power/endurance response. With moderate repetitions (6 to 15), less than 30 seconds rest between sets will key in more on muscle endurance. Rest intervals between 30 seconds and two minutes elicit strength, power, and some muscular endurance adaptations. Two-minute (or more) rest intervals target pure strength and mass gains. You'll be able to lift heavier weights with longer rest periods between sets and fewer reps per set.

Try applying "quality versus quantity" to your workouts, preferring to overload the muscle maximally each set during a shorter workout to promote strength gains and time efficiency. Most players prefer to complete a short, high-intensity workout over a long, less intense workout. For maximal overloading, use spotters to help players lift one extra rep each set.

Speed of Movement

Muscle growth is related to the amount of tension developed within the muscle. Slow-velocity lifts, which produce a great amount of tension, are used to build a base of strength and muscle mass (figure 4.1). This is why high-intensity training produces great results—on the last couple of reps, the muscle has to recruit more and more muscle fibers to keep moving the weight. There is a lot more force produced to keep the weight moving. The movement is slow, but the muscle and strength gains are fast! Slow-velocity lifts also reduce the chance for injury during weight training: Injuries are usually related to the speed of movement, not the weight.

For the hockey player who must ultimately execute fast and powerful movements, heavy weights and slow movements are first needed to develop a base of strength and lean mass; then fast movements are used

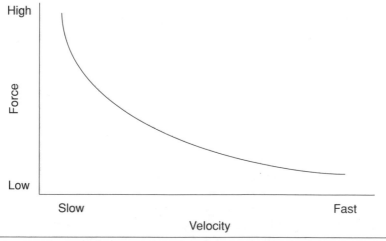

Figure 4.1 Relationship between speed of movement and force generated.

to train the nervous system and prepare the muscles for high-speed, explosive strength. Since neural adaptations are part of strength training, both the muscles and neural systems that send the messages from the brain to the muscles must be developed together so that the muscles can be trained to fire quickly.

Eccentric Contractions

During a biceps curl, when you curl the bar up toward your chest, your biceps shortens (to pull your forearm up). This is called a *concentric* muscle contraction, also known as the "positive" phase of the lift. When you lower the bar back down, your biceps lengthens. This is an *eccentric* muscle contraction, known as the "negative" phase of the exercise.

Rather than just effortlessly letting the weight drop with gravity, apply some resistance and slowly lower the bar on the way down. This will accelerate your strength and lean mass gains. As you put more effort in and *slowly* lower the bar, your biceps is still lengthening, but it is *trying* to contract, which develops a great amount of tension within the muscle.

These resistive movements are called *negatives*. Negatives make an exercise much more efficient. Why only benefit from 50 percent of the movements (the positive phase), when, by simply adding more effort to the negative (eccentric) phase, you can double your benefits?

Eccentric strength is important to hockey performance. A base of eccentric strength aids safe speed and quickness training, and high-velocity strength training. Also, eccentric strength movements are used during body contact, either while holding up your opponent, using one arm to contain an opponent who has attempted to squeeze by you, or absorbing contact along the boards. The legs are often overloaded with extreme eccentric forces when a sudden stop or sharp directional change interrupts high-speed skating. Players must have the eccentric strength to handle such abrupt stops. Eccentric strength also decreases the time it takes to absorb a sudden stop.

Following initial eccentric workouts, players will have some delayed muscle soreness. But the soreness will cease after an eccentric break-in period and a couple of full workouts. Slow-velocity movements, high-intensity, high-tension, maximal overload—all of these produce the greatest strength gains and muscle growth, and all are accomplished with negatives.

Muscle Balance

Another component of the "base of strength," muscle balance means having comparable strength in opposing muscle groups—for example, in the hamstrings (back of the upper leg) and the opposing quadriceps (thigh area). Muscle balance is important, as it reduces the possibility of a quick contraction of a strong muscle resulting in a tear of a weak opposing muscle. When developing a strength training program, make sure to include exercises for all major muscle groups, adding more exercises to improve weaker groups.

A balance of strength in each leg is important. If, as a defenseman, your left leg is stronger, you'll tend to favor it. When backing up (gliding) on the ice, you'll have more of your body weight on the left side. If you must suddenly cut laterally to the left to cut off an opposing forward, there is a delay before you can explode to the left because you must first shift more weight over to the right leg so you can push off to the left! This very brief delay will result in losing one-on-ones and races for loose pucks.

During linear acceleration, you'll get a strong pushoff with the left leg, but the right will not generate as much force against the ice to equally propel the body forward. The right will be a weaker stride, which alters technique and wastes valuable time. You will not continue accelerating at the same rate until you can plant the left foot back under your body for another powerful pushoff.

Muscle imbalances in players can pose a special problem for coaches attempting to evaluate players. In both examples above, it would be difficult to pinpoint the player's strength discrepancy with the naked eye. The coach would likely label the player as "slow." When the defenseman could not cut to the left quick enough, the coach might assume the problem is poor skating technique or poor agility. The defenseman may have the capacity for efficient skating technique, quickness, and agility, yet a simple strength imbalance prevents the proper execution of the skating techniques and prevents the player from remaining in a balanced, ready position for immediate explosive acceleration.

There are many underlying components to quick and agile skating movements. Coaches must be thorough when evaluating players; they must break down skills to their component parts so appropriate developmental programs can be structured. Basic strength tests can be useful for the coach to assess readiness for skill and technique learning, as well as for speed, quickness, and agility instruction.

To correct strength imbalances, George Nevole, conditioning coach at Cornell University, recommends training "down" to the weaker side in the weight room. If one hamstring is weaker than the other, for example, do alternate single-leg sets with the same weight based on the weaker leg. The stronger leg will maintain strength, and eventually the weak leg will catch up.

Doug Gilmour

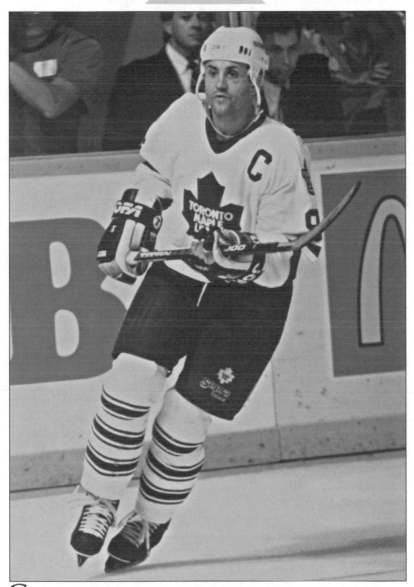

Coaches, media, and fans rave about Doug Gilmour's leadership ability. From junior hockey, where he lead the OHL in scoring, he was selected to the First All-Star team, and was named the league's MVP, to the NHL, where he was captain of the Maple Leafs and currently plays for New Jersey, Gilmour is respected as an intense competitor who thrives on the "big" games. He has played in over 1,000 NHL games, scoring over 1,000 points. He has scored at least 20 goals in 12 straight full NHL seasons and holds an NHL scoring record for notching two shorthanded goals only four seconds apart. Gilmour played for Canada at the 1990 World Championships and the 1987 Canada Cup. Like all players, there was a time when he was first introduced to conditioning and fitness testing. "At the time, I was thinking, 'Why are we doing this?' but at a later date I better understood the benefits. You practice how you play, and the harder you practice, the harder you play. I truly believe that. Obviously, your commitment to conditioning and preparation determines how hard you play. The better conditioned you are, the harder you practice, and the longer you can practice. The harder and longer you practice, the better player and team you become. And the more you practice the better conditioned you become, so it is a circular relationship—but it should all start with conditioning."

The 1992-93 season highlighted Gilmours' commitment to both ends of the rink. His offensive achievements included setting the Leaf's record for most points in a season (127) and finishing second in overall league scoring. He won the Frank J. Selke Trophy for the NHL's top defensive forward the very same year. This well-rounded ability was recognized when he finished second in voting for the league MVP. This type of achievement takes hard work, as does success in any field. I asked Doug if he had any general advice for parents and their children. "The biggest thing for the parents is to try and tell their kids exactly what it takes if they want to be a professional athlete—but to let the kids have fun, too. For the kids, they should go out and have fun, but they have to go out and have fun by working hard. Whether it's hockey or life or school or a job— whatever they want to be and whatever they want to do, they've got to work very hard and condition their mind to achieving it."

Equipment

When developing a strength training program, you'll want to choose equipment that maximizes transferability and efficiency and prevents injury.

Machines Versus Free Weights

Weight machines typically isolate one muscle group. Resistance comes from either a pin-selected weight stack, or by loading weight plates. Many strength machines can help develop a base of strength; they are also good for building up a specific muscle group to balance an opposing muscle group. Machines are also valuable in allowing a player to complete strength rehabilitation workouts while injured.

However, you do not play hockey sitting with your weight supported (as you do on most strength machines), performing isolated, re-stricted, single-plane movements with just your arms (or legs). Because hockey involves multijoint movements and a lot of single-leg activity, free weights are better than machines to prepare players for game demands. Free weights also allow for more specific and complex exercises.

Players should use multijoint exercises like the squat, a variety of lunges, and cleans. These exercises use several joints, many joint angles, and take the muscles through a full range of motion, developing balance, stability, acceleration and deceleration capabilities, and both primary and stabilizing muscles.

A machine that can build strength and power and has immediate transfer to on-ice skating is called Speedtraxx (see page 92). With Speedtraxx stride exercises a single leg must balance the body in a deep knee-bend position, while the other leg pushes off in a movement pattern similar to the skating stride using the same muscles. The leg is outwardly rotated, and the angles at the hip, knee, and ankle joints duplicate on-ice skating. The foot and leg are at a 45-degree angle to the direction of travel, just as in forward skating. The ankle and leg are at a 45-degree angle to the floor, just as on the ice when accelerating, stopping, or crossing over.

Weightlifting Belts

Many fitness and strength training books recommend wearing a weight belt for safety. I do *not* allow athletes to wear belts. If they're concerned that their backs cannot handle an exercise, they should not artificially support the back and abdominal muscles with a weight belt. Rather, they should lower the weight, spend time refining their technique, add eccentrics to help overload the muscles with less weight, or most often, add supplemental exercises to strengthen the back and abdominals until their muscles are developed enough to support the exercise. Relying on a belt in the weight room does not help a player who has to move a 220-pound opponent on the ice. Build up the back and abdominal strength—do not compensate for inadequate torso strength or poor technique with a weight belt.

Weight belts *should* be worn, however, when attempting a maximal or near maximal lift for an exercise that places a lot of stress on the lower back. But I do not recommend athletes use super heavy weights or attempt 1-RM lifts with exercises that put a lot of stress on their lower backs.

Breathing

Holding your breath while lifting a weight can cause increased blood pressure and pose potential heart problems. The high blood pressure can cause you to feel dizzy or faint (not a good situation while holding a weight!).

The common instruction for breathing during strength training is to *exhale* on the positive phase of the lift (the difficult portion—for example, when curling the bar up during a biceps curl) and to *inhale* during the negative phase (the easy portion—for example, lowering the bar in the negative phase of a biceps curl). This instruction is often incorrect, as it assumes you are exerting effort to lift the bar and then just letting the bar lower with gravity. Giving resistance on the negative phase requires a lot more effort, and a lot more tension is developed in the muscle. It's better to exhale during *both* effort phases and to pause briefly at the top and bottom for inhalation. For more explosive exercise lifts, breathe out during the positive phase and inhale during the negative phase.

OFF-ICE STRENGTH EXERCISES
TOTAL BODY

POWERCLEANS

Focus: A total body exercise: legs, hips, back, arms, trapezius

Procedure: Squatting, grasp the bar with a shoulder-width overhand grip, arms outside your knees. Position your shoulders over the bar and maintain a flat back. Begin the upward movement by extending your knees, moving your hips forward. Keep the bar close to your body throughout the lift. Keep pulling the bar up the quadriceps, then explosively extend your ankles, knees, and hip in a jumping movement. At the end of the jump phase, shrug your shoulders and pull up with your arms, leading with your elbows. To finish, rotate your elbows around and under the bar, rack the bar on the front of your shoulders, and lower your hips and knees to absorb the weight.

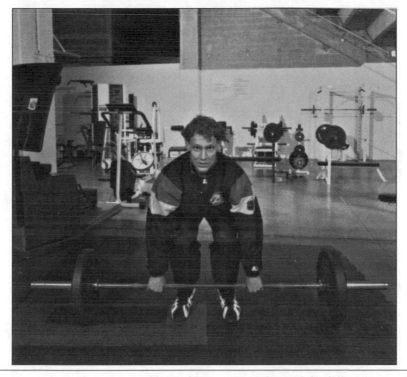

The powerclean (demonstrated by Jyrki Lumme on this and the following page) requires movement through the entire body to execute and helps on the ice with body checks, contact along the boards, and explosive acceleration.

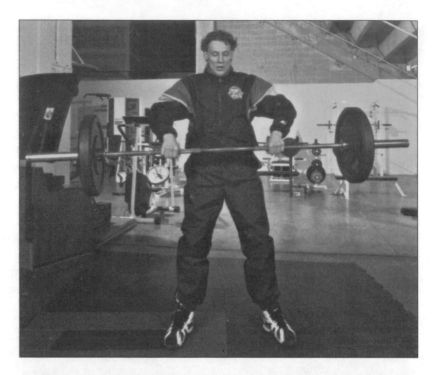

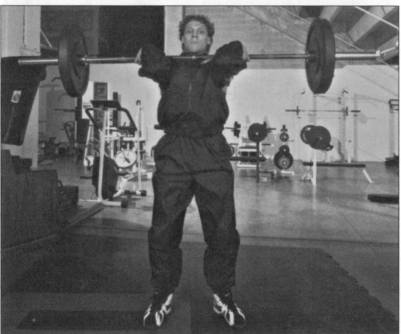

TORSO

GOODMORNINGS

Focus: Lower back

Procedure: Stand upright with an empty bar across your shoulders and
knees slightly bent. Slowly bend forward at the waist, keeping your
back straight and head up. Young athletes can initiate this exercise
using a hockey stick across their shoulders.

TRUNK ROLLS

Focus: Abdominals and back

Procedure: Player lies on floor (preferably cushioned mat), with legs
straight out along ground and arms straight out on ground over head.
Player lifts feet slightly off ground, and holds light medicine ball in
hands. Player rolls left down mat, then returns rolling right. The key
is to try to keep feet very slightly off ground and ball (hands) slightly
off ground while rolling.

WEIGHT PLATE STICKHANDLING

Focus: Abdominals, low back

Procedure: Stand upright with your knees slightly flexed. Hold a
hockey stick upside down, placing the end in the hole of an Olympic
plate. Slowly move the plate through a wide figure-8 movement.
Then move the plate left to right, moving it as wide outside the body
as possible.

FULL BENT-LEG SIT-UPS

Focus: Abdominals

Procedure: Lie on your back with your knees flexed to 90 degrees and
your feet flat on the floor. Place your hands at the side of your head.
Ankles are *not* held. Likewise, do not pull behind your head. Slowly
sit up, using only your abdominals, until your elbows touch the
knees. Lower under control, taking the same time to lower as it did to
sit up.

CRUNCHES

Focus: Abdominals

Procedure: Lie on your back, knees flexed to 90 degrees and feet in the air. Place your hands at the side of your head. "Crunch" your abdominals together, curling your elbows toward your knees and pulling your knees up and in toward your head. Meet in the middle and slowly lower back to the starting position.

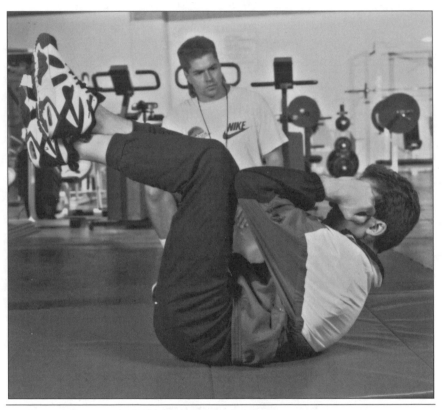

Tim Hunter demonstrates proper crunch positioning.

LOWER AB PUSH PRESS

Focus: Lower abdominals

Procedure: Lie on your back with your legs straight up in the air, feet together. Place your hands on the floor under your buttocks. Using your lower abdominals, push your legs toward the ceiling. Think of pushing the bottom of your feet toward the ceiling. Your legs move straight up and down by moving your hips two to six inches in the air.

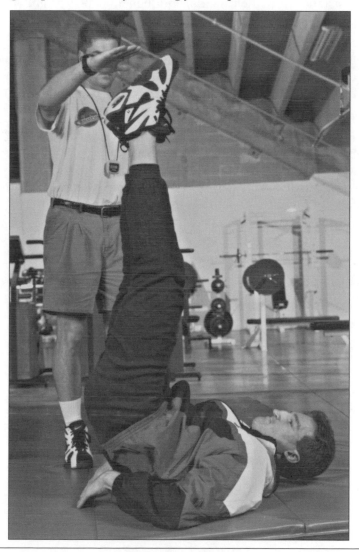

Conditioning coach Pete Twist gives Tim Hunter a target to push his feet up toward during the lower abdominal push press.

Coaching Tips:

1. The difficulty of this exercise will amaze most players. You only need to move two to six inches. Due to an overreliance on curl-ups and crunches, most athletes will be unable to do this exercise with strict technique. To begin, allow athletes to get a small pushoff from their hands underneath their gluteals, or a small leg-swing, to assist the movement. These serve as a "self-spot." Once their lower abs begin to develop, keep technique strict. No pushoff assistance from their hands, and legs must be upright and completely stationary prior to each rep.

2. Even if they can do this exercise without assistance, they will still feel they need to force out a longer range of movement, and will ultimately cheat and alter technique to move their feet higher in the air. Reassure players that a small range of motion is correct for this exercise.

3. Instruct players to really focus on using their lower abs to initiate the movement.

4. Always perform lower abdominal exercises first. Since the upper abdominals assist with movements for the lower abdominals, fatigued upper abdominals interfere with completion of lower abdominal exercises.

UPPER BODY

LAT PULL-DOWNS

Focus: Back

Procedure: Keeping your torso erect, grasp the bar with a wide over-hand grip. Pull down to the back of your neck, keeping your neck as straight as possible. Raise the bar as high as you can, under control

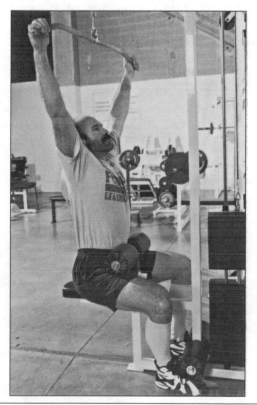

Dave Babych shows starting position of the lat pull-down exercise.

SEATED ROWS

Focus: Back

Procedure: Sit down with your back straight and your knees slightly bent. Grasp the bar with a closed grip. Pull the bar from your foot area in toward your lower chest area. In the contracted position, your back should be straight and your shoulders rotated back. Think of squeezing your shoulder blades together at the finish position. When lowering the bar, let your torso lean forward slightly, but initiate the next pull with your upper back and arms, not your lower back.

BENCH PRESS

Focus: Chest, shoulders, triceps

Procedure: Lie on the bench and grasp the bar with a wide overhand grip. Slowly lower the bar to the midchest region, and then push the bar up on a slight arc back to the starting position. Keep your feet flat on the floor and your back flat on the bench throughout the exercise.

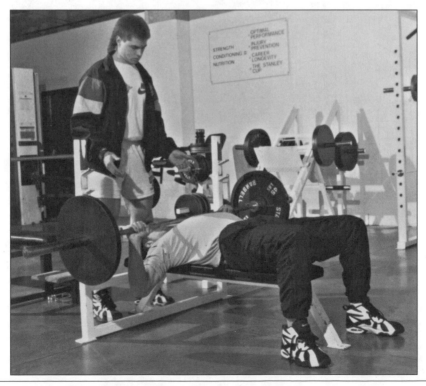

Pete Twist spots Bret Hedican on the bench press exercise.

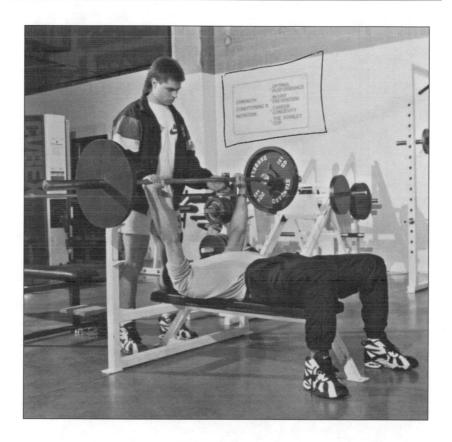

DUMBBELL FLYS

Focus: Chest

Procedure: Lie face up on a bench with your back flat and your feet flat on the floor (see photos on next page). Begin with dumbbells up above your chest, the palms of your hands facing inward. With a slight elbow flexion, slowly lower the dumbbells in an arc, lowering your elbows toward the floor until you feel a good stretch in the chest and shoulders. Push the dumbbells back up until your arms are fully extended over the top of your chest. To achieve the proper arc, think of hugging a barrel.

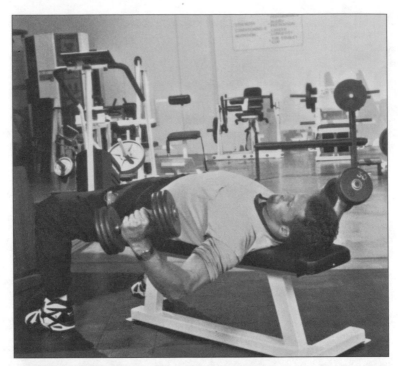

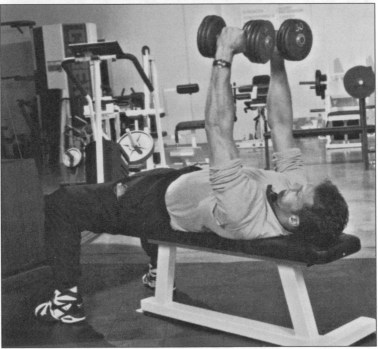

Bret Hedican completes dumbbell flys.

MEDICINE BALL CHEST PASS (LONG DISTANCE)

Focus: Chest, shoulders, triceps

Procedure: Stand with knees slightly bent, shoulder-width stance, 9 to 12 feet from a partner. Hold your hands out in front of your chest for a target. Catch and absorb your partner's pass, bringing the ball into your chest, and immediately extend your arms out to pass the ball back to your partner. After you pass off, keep your arms extended and your hands up, ready to receive the pass back.

PUSH PRESS

Focus: Shoulders, triceps

Procedure: Stand upright, holding a bar on the front of your shoulders with a shoulder-width overhand grip. Drop your hips a few inches, and drive your legs back up, following through by pushing the bar upward until you fully extend your arms over your head. Lower the bar under control back to your shoulders. Be careful not to arch your back.

LATERAL RAISES

Focus: Shoulders

Procedure: Stand upright with your knees slightly bent, holding dumbbells at your sides. Lift the dumbbells up and out at your sides until the dumbbells are higher than your shoulders. Slowly lower the dumbbells back to your sides.

UPRIGHT ROWS

Focus: Shoulders, trapezius

Procedure: Stand upright with your knees slightly flexed, grasping the bar with an overhand grip, hands four to eight inches apart. Leading with your elbows, pull the bar upward along the abdominals and chest toward your chin. At the top of the pull, your elbows are higher than your wrists and above your shoulders. Lower the bar under control.

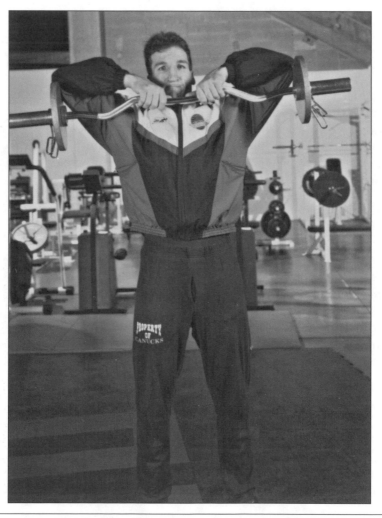

Tim Hunter performing upright rows.

ARMS

LYING TRICEPS EXTENSIONS

Focus: Triceps

Procedure: Lie flat on a bench with your feet flat on the floor. Grasp an EZ-curl bar with a close overhand grip. Start with the bar above the top of your head, lower under control just past your forehead (so that if you dropped the bar, it would fall over your head). Push the bar back up on an arc until your arms are fully extended. Throughout the lift your elbows should remain stationary and be kept close together.

DIPS

Focus: Triceps, shoulders, chest

Procedure: Grasp the dip bars with your arms fully extended and your knees flexed. Keeping your torso upright, slowly lower your body until your arms are flexed and your chest is even with the dip bars. Push back up until your arms are fully extended.

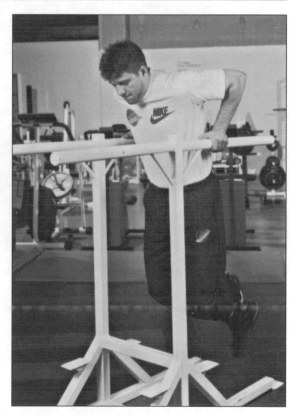

Alek Stojanov completes a set of dips.

STANDING BARBELL CURLS

Focus: Biceps

Procedure: Grasp a bar with a shoulder-width underhand grip. Stand upright with your knees slightly flexed. Start with the bar resting in front of the quadriceps. Pull the bar up in an arc by flexing your arms at the elbows. Select a weight you can lift without arching your back or swinging your hips into the lift. Lower the bar slowly under control.

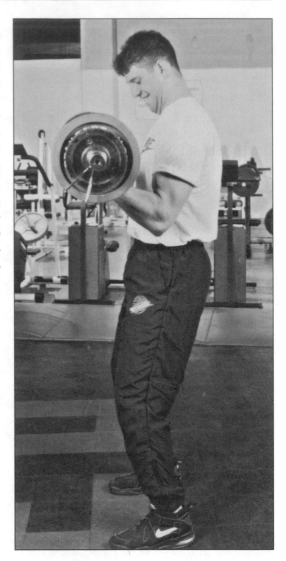

Alek Stojanov shows proper technique with standing barbell curls.

HAMMER CURLS

Focus: Outer biceps, forearms

Procedure: Stand upright with your knees slightly flexed, holding dumbbells with an overhand grip. Start with the dumbbells resting at your side, palms turned in toward the outer side of your legs. Maintain your hand position, lifting the dumbbells up in an arc to chest height by flexing at the elbows. Slowly lower, keeping your elbows at your sides. Select a weight you can lift without swinging your arms.

REVERSE CURLS

Focus: Forearms, wrists

Procedure: Grasp a bar with a shoulder-width overhand grip. Stand upright with your knees slightly flexed. Start with the bar resting in front of the quadriceps. Pull the bar up in an arc by flexing your arms at the elbows and directing the back of your hands toward the shoulders. Select a weight you can lift without swinging your hips into the lift. Lower the bar slowly under control.

WRIST CURLS

Focus: Wrists, forearms

Procedure: Sit on a bench and position one arm so that your forearm is resting flat on the bench with your wrist just over the edge of the bench, the palm of your hand facing up. Holding a dumbbell, slowly roll the dumbbell down your hand until held by your fingertips. Curl the dumbbell back up, flexing at the wrist. Complete the same exercise with your palms facing down, curling the wrist up and down.

WRIST ROTATIONS

Focus: Wrists, forearms

Procedure: Sit on a bench and position one arm so that your forearm is resting flat on the bench with your wrist just over the edge of the bench. Hold one end of a small bar that is weighted at one end. Twist your forearm left and right in a controlled fashion.

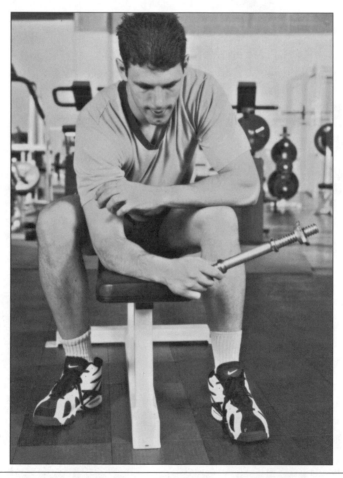

Wrist rotations, performed by Gino Odjick, build forearm strength.

LOWER BODY

SQUATS

Focus: Legs, gluteals, back

Procedure: Stand upright with bar balanced on back using a wide overhand grip. Feet should be shoulder-width apart and parallel, with toes pointed out slightly. Maintaining a straight back, with your head up, focus your eyes on a point slightly higher than head level. Begin to lower the weight by dropping the hips into a seated position and flexing the knees. Your weight should be on the middle to back of the feet. Your knees should remain over your feet—if you glance down they should never be out past your toes. Lower until your quadriceps are parallel to the ground, then raise the bar by straightening the hips and knees.

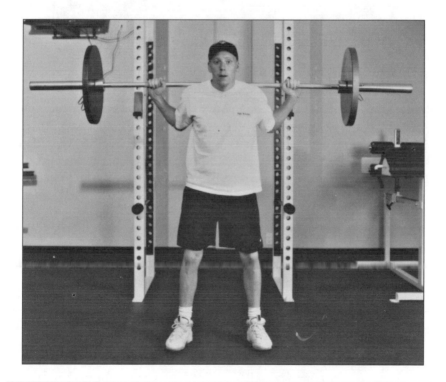

Corey Hirsch shows proper squat positioning on this and the following page. Technique should be assessed by viewing from the front, rear, and side.

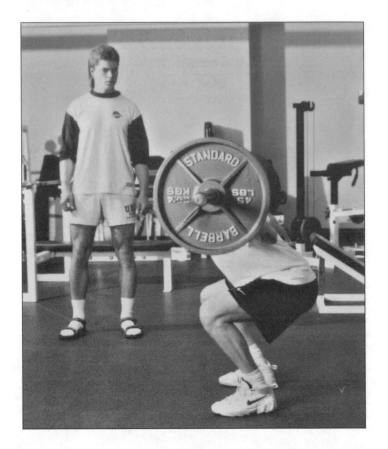

Many coaches will say that squats are dangerous. Players have told me, "I used to do squats, but they hurt my knees." The truth is squats build up strength around your knees. *Incorrect* squats can hurt your knees, and hockey can tear down your knees, but correct squats build up your knee strength. I actually use controlled squats and partial squats only days after players suffer certain serious knee ligament injuries in a game. Squats are very safe. *Any* exercise done incorrectly is dangerous. Inevitably, all players claiming hurt knees demonstrate similar incorrect technique. They initiate their descent at the knees, and end up with their weight on their toes and their knees out past their toes, putting most of the force on their knees! Start lowering into a squat by first lowering your buttocks, like sitting onto a chair. In the squat, your weight should be on your heels—you should be able to move your toes up off the ground while in the squat position. Your knees should remain over your toes—never out in front of them. You'll feel a little off balance the first few times you try the correct technique. Soon it will feel natural, and you'll be on your way to safely developing some important skating muscles.

SEATED LEG CURLS

Focus: Hamstrings

Procedure: Sit upright and curl the weight down by flexing at the knees. Keep your back flat against the back rest.

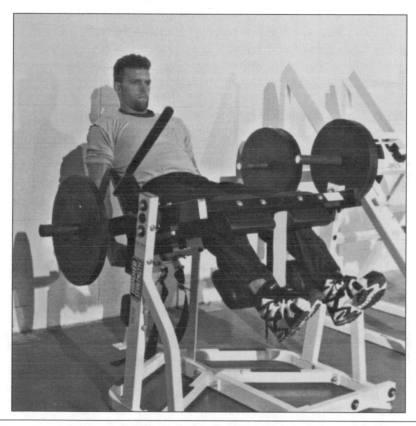

The seated leg curl, demonstrated by Bret Hedican, develops hamstring strength.

WALKING LUNGES

Focus: Hamstrings, quadriceps, groin, gluteals, calves, hip extensors, hip flexors

Procedure: Standing up straight, step out with one leg as far as you can, plant foot on ground heel first, and roll onto foot as you lower the hips and buttocks toward the ground. As with squats, your front knee should never end up out in front of your toes. If it is, your stride is too short. Start again and lengthen your stride. From start to finish, keep the torso in an upright position, back straight. After you land on the left leg, push off with the right, bringing the body upright and follow through by stepping forward with the right leg. Continue stepping forward and lunging, alternating legs down the floor. Beginners will need time to progress into the stride length and depth of hips in the finishing position. When beginning lunges, even if you have a great base of strength, complete no more than a total of 30 repetitions. Lunge exercises, which target the skating muscles and work a lot of muscles at once, require good balance and are a great single-leg exercise. But they also have a great potential for delayed muscle soreness after the first two or three lunge workouts.

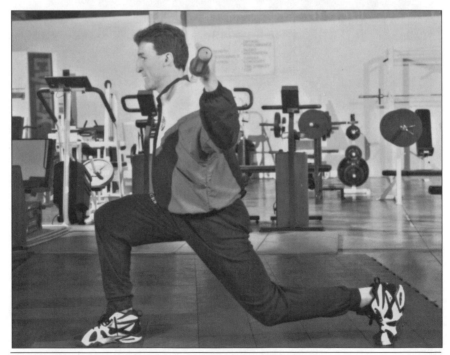

Tim Hunter shows good technique in the lunge.

HOCKEY LUNGES

Focus: Hamstrings, quadriceps, groin, gluteals, calves, abductors, hip extensors, hip flexors

Procedure: These are similar to walking lunges, but you stride out at a 45-degree angle (an angle similar to the push-off on the ice), with your leg outwardly rotated and your body weight over this single striding leg, just like on the ice. When landing, the foot should be in line with the leg to protect your knee—if the foot faces forward when it plants, there will be irregular stress placed sideways on the knee. Planting the foot in line with the leg (out at a 45-degree angle) also puts that leg in a position to push off the next stride at a 45-degree angle. In the photo, Tim Hunter lunges out at a 45-degree angle, landing on his left foot. He will immediately push off with the right foot, moving his body weight over the left foot where he is ready to push off to the opposite side at a 45-degree angle, where he will plant his right foot to land.

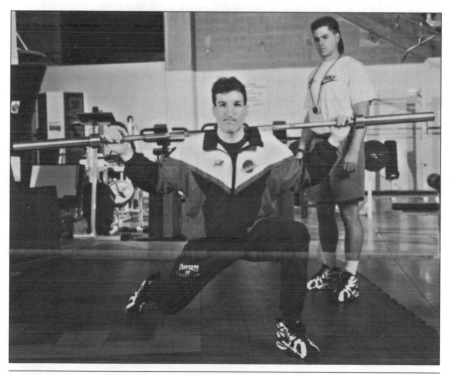

Tim Hunter striding through a set of hockey lunges.

SUMO SIDE LUNGES

Focus: Hamstrings, quadriceps, groin, gluteals, abductors

Procedure: These are a combination of squats and lunges. Step out to the right and squat, push back to your starting stance. Step out to the left and lower to a one-leg squat, push back to your starting stance. Use no weight or a light weight with this exercise. Too much weight is risky because of the single-leg support position, the stress on the groin, and because the sideways step places some lateral stress on the knee—a type of strength you need to build, but a movement that becomes higher risk when accompanied by excessive weight. Technique and function is most important here—not the amount of weight used. I recommend using, at most, an empty 45-pound bar for this exercise. Also, as with squats and lunges, watch the position of the knee relative to the foot.

SPEEDTRAXX HOCKEY STRIDE

Focus: Hip extensors, quadriceps, gluteals, abductors, hamstrings, groin

Procedure: Position the left track at 45 degrees. Place your support foot up close to the machine base, and grasp the support handles (see photo on the next page). Place the toes of your left foot on the track pedal, the ankle in the air at an angle. Drop your hips and stay as low as you can on the support leg while you push off with your left leg to full extension. Exaggerate your stride to as long a push as possible. The lower you are able to stay on your support leg, the longer stride you will achieve. Repeat this for a set with your right leg. (*Note:* Once this movement is comfortable, try to stride off without hanging on to the handles. These "free-standing strides" turn it into a free-weight, multijoint type exercise and places more emphasis on your abdominals, back, and gluteals as the stabilizing point, as opposed to leveraging off of your hand support.)

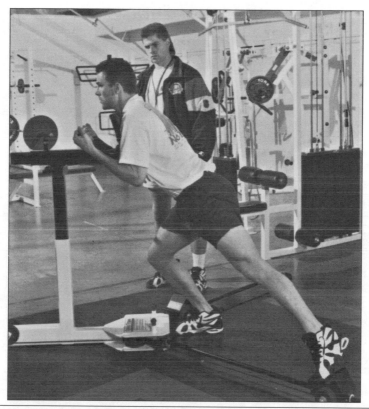

Trevor Linden builds up strength and power in his left leg for his hockey stride, while developing single-leg balance and strength in his right leg.

SPEEDTRAXX CROSSOVER STRIDE

Focus: Groin, quadriceps

Procedure: For this exercise, one track is set in a linear, straight position. Position your body sideways to the machine (see photo on the next page). Lean on the pad, with one arm over the pad. Place your support foot over the track and your stride foot on the track pedal. Push off along the track until full leg extension. This is similar to the inside skate pushoff when crossing over around a corner.

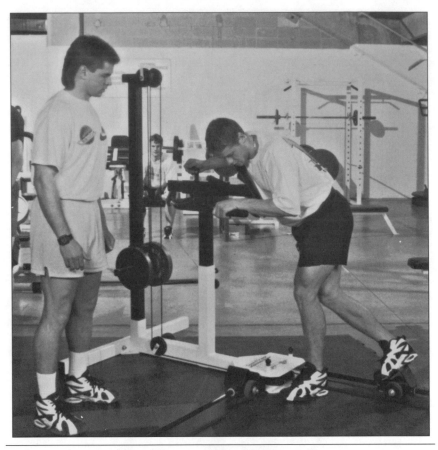

Pavel Bure works at the Speedtraxx crossover stride exercise.

LATERAL CROSSOVER BOX STEP-UPS

Focus: Gluteals, hamstrings, quadriceps, groin, abductors

Procedure: Standing away from and sideways to a stable box, complete a Sumo Side Lunge to step in closer to the box (see photos on the next page). With your outside leg, step over the inside leg right up onto the box. Pushing off with your foot that remains on the ground, bring the inside leg up on the box. Try to keep your shoulders and hips facing square throughout this movement to really challenge your flexibility around the hips. Use a very light weight and take as long a stride as possible—really exaggerate your range of movement.

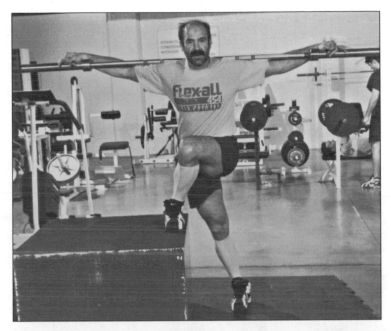

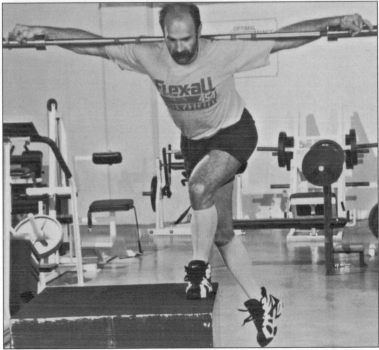

Dave Babych developed these lateral crossover box step-ups to complement a series of lateral strength, quickness, and agility exercises and drills.

SPEEDTRAXX LATERAL STRIDE

Focus: Abductors, adductors (groin)

Procedure: Position one track in a direct lateral position. Place your support foot up close to the machine base, or even up on top of the base. Drop the hips and stay as low as possible. With your other leg, push off in a direct lateral position to full leg extension.

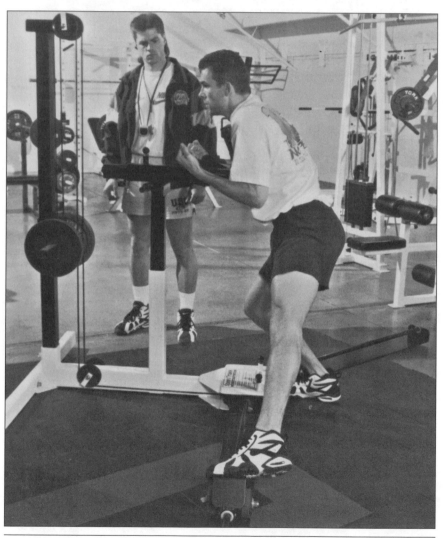

A set of Speedtraxx lateral strides is completed by Trevor Linden.

ABDUCTION/ADDUCTION

Focus: Abductors, adductors (groin)

Procedure: Stand facing the total hip machine. Lift your right leg up and out to the side, flexing at the knee. Position the pad roller inside your right leg. Using your adductors, bring the roller down toward your body. Next, lift your knee up and across your body. Position the pad roller on the outside of your leg. Using your abductors, push the pad away from your body, out to the side. Repeat sets for your other leg. You can also try this exercise with surgical tubing.

HIP FLEXION/HIP EXTENSION

Focus: Hip flexors, hip extensors

Procedure: Stand sideways to the total hip machine. Place the roller above the knee of your inside leg. Lift your knee up as high as possible. Next, lift your knee up and position the roller behind the knee. Drive the roller down and behind your body. Repeat with your other leg. You can also do this exercise with surgical tubing.

ON-ICE STRENGTH EXERCISES

EXAGGERATED CROSSOVERS AROUND A CIRCLE

Focus: Quadriceps, hamstrings, gluteals, abductors, adductors (groin), hip flexors, hip extensors

Procedure: Slowly skate around a circle. Drop your hips as low as possible, cross over, and lengthen your inside crossover stride as far as possible. Keep the knee of the support leg flexed as you move slowly through this lengthened stride.

LONG LATERAL CROSSOVERS

Focus: Hamstrings, quadriceps, groin, gluteals, abductors, adductors (groin)

Procedure: Step into a Sumo Side Lunge, then follow through crossing right over the inside leg. Make the Sumo Side Lunge as wide as possible, lower your hips as far as possible, and exaggerate the crossover step.

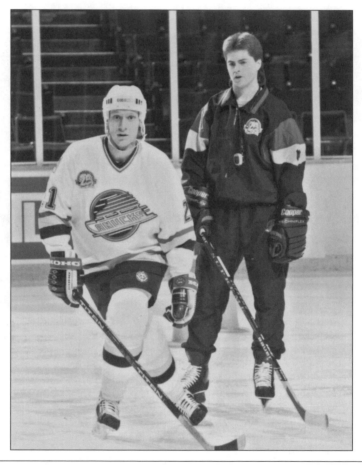

Jyrki Lumme demonstrates the long lateral crossover. Step laterally with as wide a step as you can, keeping your hips low, then rise up and cross over.

RESISTED FORWARD PIVOTS

Focus: All skating muscles

Procedure: The player's coach or partner provides skating resistance by holding a belt or tubing that trails behind the skater. Set up pylons on a 45-degree angle from each other, so the player is moving side to side down the ice. The coach holds the belt and glides straight down the ice, in the middle of the pylons, while the player takes strong powerful strides to skate around each pylon.

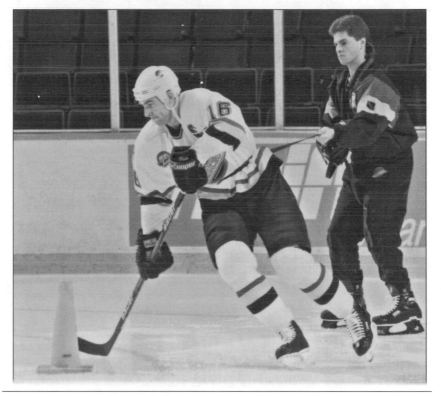

Trevor Linden goes through the resisted forward pivot drill on this and the following page. This is a great drill for forcing players to focus on driving the legs and fighting through checks.

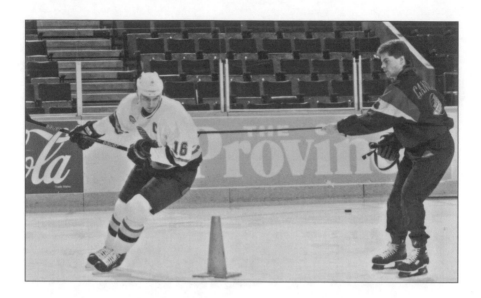

ON-ICE WALKING LUNGES

Focus: Hamstrings, quadriceps, groin, gluteals, calves, hip flexors, hip extensors

Procedure: Complete these the same as dry-land walking lunges. You will need to slow your movement down to prevent too much gliding action. Be sure to elongate your stride and lower the hips as far as possible.

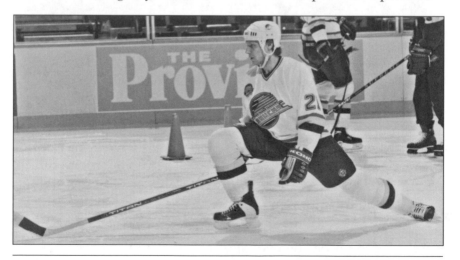

Jyrki Lumme pushes off with his left leg and keeps his weight balanced over his right leg during a set of on-ice walking lunges.

CHAPTER 5

QUICKNESS AND AGILITY TRAINING

Although Pavel Bure obviously has good speed, he is *not* the fastest hockey player I've coached. I've coached college athletes who are faster. I can say this with confidence, pointing to the definitions of *speed* and *quickness*. I measure how fast athletes skate by their linear acceleration and maximum speed. These qualities are important when you're dumping the puck in and forechecking, for instance, or when you're racing down the ice to determine an icing call. But far more often than pure speed, the hockey player draws upon quickness and agility. *Quickness* is the first-step explosion from a stationary position. It is reacting and exploding into action. Coaches have forever dreamed of players with "explosive speed"—this is quickness.

Hockey is a game of one-on-one battles and races for loose pucks. The ability to *initiate* movement faster than opponents is critical—teams rarely lose if they are consistently the first to the puck and always right on top of the play. Although members of the media marvel at Pavel's speed, the Russian Rocket's explosiveness is fueled by quickness. His quickness is so great that he can be at his top speed in just two or three strides. Other players may be faster, but they take the whole length of the ice before they reach their top speed. In a controlled test, others may win a race of one complete lap of the ice, but if they take a half-lap to reach top speed, this is of little value in a game. Pavel wins races for loose pucks not because of his speed but because of his incredible quickness—that first-step explosiveness. He does not have the best top speed, but he reaches his top speed *first*, in a couple of strides, so he is at his top speed longer than his opponents. Pavel is at his top speed while others are still just initiating movement.

Alex Mogilny is able to accomplish explosiveness while handling the puck—a skill that slows many players down. Both Pavel and Alex are

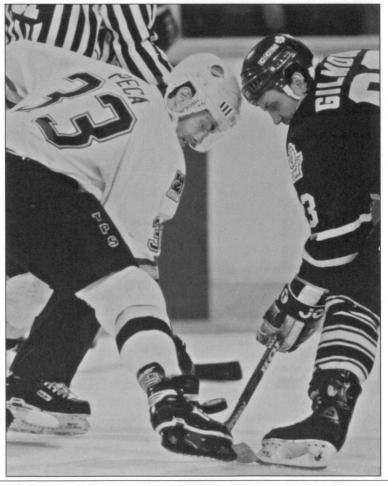

Winning a face-off requires explosive reactions. Here Mike Peca and Doug Gilmour position themselves for the draw.

exciting to watch skating full-out on a breakaway. But most critical game-breaking plays start with quickness. For Bure and Mogilny, being able to cut on a dime and explode two strides laterally while carrying the puck is what positioned them for the breakaway everyone notices. Murray Craven, of the Chicago Black Hawks, stresses the importance of quickness training. "Today in hockey, all players are bigger, faster, and stronger than they used to be," says Craven. "It's often quickness that separates a junior player or a minor league player from a NHL player. It's that first couple of steps to get to loose pucks, to get to the pucks in front of the net—that's what makes big goal scorers these days."

As a defenseman, the Canucks' Bret Hedican epitomizes quickness when he quarterbacks the play out of his end, attacking right to the opposition's net. If the play does not result in a goal, Bret will be the first player back to our net. He explodes so quickly to his top skating speed that he really gets a jump on his opponents, and he can also cover for himself if pulled out of position. Quickness affords young players room for error while they refine their decision making for defensive responsibilities, positioning, and coverage.

Quickness is also invaluable when a player is skating down the ice at or near top speed. During a one-on-one, full-out speed is easy for a defenseman to stay with and contain—because it is *predictable* and the defenseman simply adjusts his backward skating speed and his angles relative to the speed of the oncoming forward.

But if a forward is sprinting down the wing, and, when getting close to the defenseman, can instantaneously adjust his speed, rapidly alternating between decelerating and accelerating, the defenseman is challenged to continually read and react to cover the forward. When the forward sees the defenseman shift his weight in trying to react to the forward's quick change in speed (decelerating), the forward can then explode to the highest speed and move around the defenseman. The ability to quickly change speed while already skating fast is very effective for throwing off a defender. Being able to shift from fourth gear down to third and jump back up to fifth in the blink of an eye is one of *the* most dangerous offensive tools.

Quickness is also useful, combined with strength, during open-ice bodychecks. Perfectly executed, these are one of the most beautiful hockey movements. Strength is a more obvious component of the movement, but to execute open-ice hits correctly, you have to be able to read the play, react quickly to move into position for the hit, quickly lower your body into a power position, and explosively thrust upward, first with the legs and then quickly following through with the arms. The weight transfer from low to high must be explosive to overpower an opponent who is skating the opposite direction.

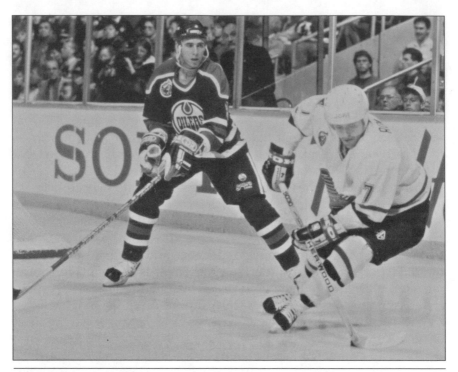

Cliff Ronning controls the puck while spinning to evade a defenseman.

The ability to evade an opponent, or likewise in a defensive position, to stay with and contain an opponent, depends on *agility*. This is Cliff Ronning's most valuable ability—stop-and-starts, quick turns, changes in direction, spinning, and zigzagging. All dynamic movements in a small area require agility, even if you're away from the play. During a sudden transition you want to be able to rapidly change your body position and direction to prepare yourself for the play.

It may involve reacting to cover a man. "I work on quickness off-ice, to get an explosive burst of speed from my first three strides, along with agility so I can quickly shift my position to always face the play," stresses Bret Hedican. "As a defenseman, I always need to keep an eye on where the puck is in the defensive zone. This means skating backward and quickly turning or using tight pivots to go with the puck. Defensemen need to be able to shift their body to pivot or turn forward and backward so they're always facing the play and the puck, or to stay with and cover their opponent." On the puck or off the puck, agility is a critical component.

Some big defensemen are often incorrectly called "slow" by fans and coaches. Given the space, these players' top speed is comparable to other players. What they may lack is quickness. However, they succeed in the league because they move so efficiently. They have great mobility and lateral movement—great *agility*. They may not appear quick or explosive, but their agility allows them to win one on-ones. Sometimes veteran defensemen will attribute their success in lieu of quickness to "experience," or "knowing where to move," or "positioning," not even realizing that their ability to move into position or knowing where to go or how to react is agility. Agility is stored motor patterns of complex movements. Each time you repeat a certain movement or situation, it is reinforced and becomes easier to do next time.

Quickness and agility, though two distinct parameters, are teamed together here because hockey is a multidirectional sport over short distances. Quickness can be thought of as the "first gear" of speed and is best represented by first-step explosiveness. When it's combined with agility, you get first-step explosiveness in a variety of complex movement patterns—forward skating, backward, lateral movement, 45-degree angles, directional changes, rotations, pivots, and complex movements that involve very rapid continual transfer from one movement into another, usually over just a few feet. Lift your arms straight out to your sides and note the distance from fingertip to fingertip. Often quickness and agility is executed within this distance. Agility requires precise control of your body. During a rapid movement, what are your feet, legs, hips, torso, and arms doing? At what angle are your ankle, knee, and hip joints? They all must work in an integrated, coordinated pattern.

Being able to combine quickness and agility is *the* most important hockey skill. During a hockey game, quickness and agility are manifested in many ways: for the draw on a face-off, to drop down and position the body to block a shot or make a save, to cross over and accelerate away from an opponent, to quickly stop and control the body to maintain a defensive position, to shoot the puck, and to deliver a bodycheck. Quickness and agility development helps less-skilled players become more skilled, and highly skilled players become even better.

Quickness and agility are neuromuscular skills that increase the adaptability, explosiveness, and precision with which players can handle their own bodies, facilitating coordinated efforts between body position, footwork, stick position, and puck control, all while reacting to constant and rapid changes in play and in position of the other 11 players on the ice. Players with these skills are able to execute complex and valuable maneuvers very quickly.

CONDITIONING FOR QUICKNESS AND AGILITY

Many coaches simply hope that their players will eventually improve quickness and agility through doing generic practice drills. Other coaches use repetitive sprints up and down the ice with stop-and-starts at each line, and they hope quickness is taken care of through these conditioning drills. As fatigue sets in, all the payers learn is how to skate slowly with flawed technique. Practice drills must be designed and structured appropriately for the muscles to learn to fire quicker and to allow the brain to learn and rehearse specific movement patterns at high speeds.

Quickness and agility training is *quality* training—not quantity. You want full-out efforts for a few strides followed by active recovery. Improvement is not a physical adaptation that requires overload but a neuromuscular adaptation that requires explosive and correct movement patterns with perfect technique. What you're increasing is the brain's ability to turn the machine on quicker.

On the ice, both quickness and speed, as well as agility, are primarily single-leg actions. Hockey itself is an independent leg activity. To prepare for this, I like to use a lot of single-leg drills or drills that

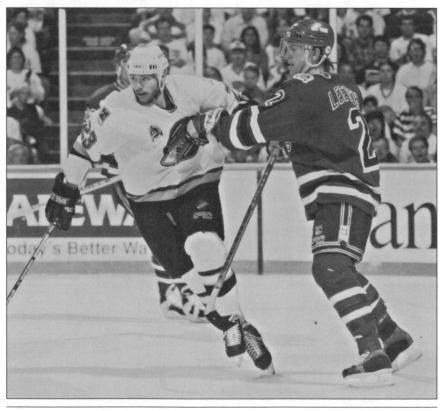

Martin Gelinas uses precise control of his entire body to receive a hit and quickly cross over and accelerate away from the defenseman, even when slightly off balance from withstanding the hit.

incorporate continual transfer from one foot to the other. On the ice, you drive off of a single leg to initiate movement. During the first three or four strides, 85 percent of your time is spent supported by one leg. In a game, you're supported on one leg the vast majority of the time. Rarely do you have your feet planted at the same time, with weight equally distributed over both feet.

Explosiveness Through Plyometrics

Plyometrics are the best type of exercises to ready the player for on-ice quickness and agility. As Jeremy Roenick notes, "For overall explosiveness, if you want to be a faster and quicker player, then plyometrics are going to be of tremendous benefit to you." These drills are characterized by jumping, hopping, bounding, and a variety of foot patterns. Plyometrics involve a rapid eccentric contraction immediately before a concentric contraction, which allows for a more powerful concentric contraction. With plyometric exercises, the muscle is rapidly loaded with an eccentric (lengthening) or negative contraction, and then immediately followed by a concentric (muscle shortening) or positive contraction, which results in a more explosive concentric contraction. You see this kind of movement during the quick backswing prior to an explosive slapshot, or the quick stop with rapid knee flexion and then immediately exploding into action in the opposite direction.

Sensors in your muscles keep track of the length of the muscle and the rate of its lengthening. If the muscle is lengthened *quickly* (e.g., when your legs bend to absorb a quick two-foot stop) your sensors detect this and tell the muscle to immediately contract to protect itself from injury. This contraction allows you to abruptly sprint out in the opposite direction. This kind of *countermovement* is common to many hockey actions and is the key component of plyometric training. The countermovement also produces potential elastic energy. When the muscle quickly lengthens, it stores elastic energy, like stretching an elastic band. If you abruptly shift to moving in the opposite direction, you harness this elastic energy for more powerful movement. However, if you slow down or pause at the bottom of the countermovement, the extra potential energy is lost as heat. Likewise, the muscle sensors no longer signal for explosive muscle action. An effective countermovement is evident when defensemen prepare for open-ice bodychecks. When approaching an opponent, just prior to the hit a defenseman will quickly drop at the hips and bend at the knees, then immediately explode in the opposite direction to deliver the bodycheck.

You can't build nonspecific strength and muscle mass and then just hope to be able to harness your increased size and strength in a game for hockey-specific, velocity-specific actions. A big, slow defenseman will not magically become explosive and agile, no matter how many times his weakness is identified and no matter how many hundreds of practices he participates in. But he *can* develop quick feet through specific training—plyometrics are a key link from strength and lean muscle mass to quickness and speed.

Plyometric *intensity* refers to the degree of impact resulting from a drill. In jumping, your joints must absorb your body weight as it lands back on the ground. This can result in a great amount of stress on the joints. The greater the jump height, the more force your ankle, knee, hip, and spine will have to endure. Also, the greater an athlete's body weight, the greater the risk of injury. Players who weigh 220 pounds develop far more stress on their joints than 170-pound players. And the lower the relative strength, the greater the risk of injury. Players who weigh 170 pounds and lack sufficient muscle development and leg strength are also at risk of injury. There is no type of exercise better at improving explosiveness than plyometrics, but there is also no exercise with a higher risk for injury.

To maximize benefits and minimize risk, use low-intensity plyometrics such as quick-feet drills, stride frequency drills, and quick-hand drills. Perform these drills in both organized and random patterns to develop hockey quickness and agility.

To ease stress on the joints, rather than relying on increased heights for jumps as a progression, try the following:

1. Increase foot quickness by "popping" your feet off the ground. Like a game of hot potatoes, as soon as the foot starts to touch the ground, pop it back off again. Pop off from the *toes*. Try to increase the number of foot contacts you can make in a set amount of time.

2. Practice quickly reversing movement and exploding in the opposite direction.

3. Eliminate the pause that occurs at the exact point where the direction of movement is going to reverse. A pause between lowering and pushing off will lose the potential elastic energy and turn off the muscle sensors, detracting from the potential power and explosiveness of the pushoff.

4. Instead of increasing vertical distances, increase both lateral and linear horizontal distances.

5. Add more complex movements (various foot patterns, rotations, angles, and turns).

6. Complete some of the lateral drills with a single leg.

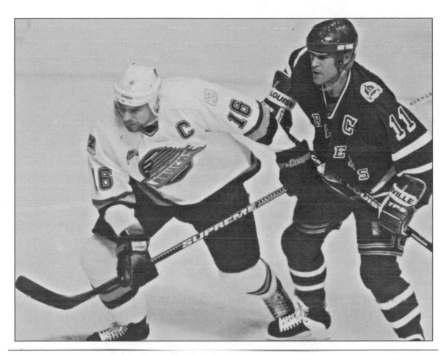

While warding off a New York Ranger with his left arm, Trevor Linden uses stride power developed by stride exercises to accelerate and avoid a crosscheck.

QUICKNESS AND AGILITY CONDITIONING GUIDELINES

Use these guidelines for a safe and effective approach to conditioning for quickness and agility:

1. At all ages and all levels, teach agility before quickness. Begin with simple movement patterns and don't increase foot speed until technique is perfect.

2. At young ages, agility is more movement specific than sport specific. Incorporate a wide variety of drills to develop a general base of athleticism and to coordinate the body in many dynamic movement patterns. Agility drills are not taxing on the joints or muscles like quickness and speed work is, so they are suitable for young athletes.

3. If the athlete has sufficient muscle mass, strength, and technique, begin to increase the explosiveness. The strength base criteria for low-intensity plyometric readiness is squatting your own body

weight. Prior to upper-body quickness drills, players should at least be able to bench press their body weight.

Readiness for high-intensity plyometrics (heights over 15 inches or hopping for distance) used to be tested by the ability to squat 1.5 times your body weight. Coaches should try having players complete a four- to six-week strength program before participating in explosive drills. They should monitor each athlete day to day through a variety of exercises to assess their readiness, rather than placing them in a single controlled test of strength. During this time coaches can informally check players' coordination, muscle balance, and strength improvements.

4. Always maintain a ready position with knees flexed and hips low. If you have to move into the ready position before you're set to accelerate, you'll suffer a critical delay in initiating the required movement.

5. Move to more hockey-specific movement patterns as development improves: lateral movement, backward, outward hip rotation, crossovers, and so on.

6. Perform at full effort until neuromuscular fatigue. Do not seek to induce physical fatigue. When fatigued, your explosiveness slows and technique falters—you'll end up practicing the incorrect movement slowly. Instead, athletes should rapidly complete precise movements so their neuromuscular system learns to organize high-velocity movements. Likewise, rest intervals must be long enough that the player does not begin any repetition in a prefatigued state.

7. Incorporate visual stimulus as players improve. This may involve catching tennis balls or receiving a pass during complex movements. Keep this part of the drill constant so players always know where to go and when a ball or puck is to come.

8. Incorporate visual or auditory stimulus in varied movement patterns. Players may explode into action after a ball is dropped in front of them in order to catch it before it hits the ground again. You may also call out directions. These are *react and explode* drills—players have to react and, with controlled movement, quickly explode or cut to a certain direction.

9. Limit initial quickness and agility drill repetitions to 5 seconds. This will help key on the explosive initiation of movement and the quality of movement. As players develop, increase to 10 or 15 seconds.

10. In a game, explosive agility may be required at the end of a shift when the athlete is fatigued, so the final progression for improved game situation agility is developing the ability to execute explosive, skillful movements in a fatigued state. To do this, I have players perform an exhausting task for 15 to 30 seconds, followed immediately by a quickness and agility drill. This helps them learn to mobilize motor units to coordinate explosive complex movements when fatigued. You still must use long work-to-rest ratios to develop quickness and agility, but once you have improved, you need to practice within game conditions.

There are hundreds of on-ice and off-ice quickness and agility drills. Many of them are fun to do. Players work hard at these drills. They compete intensely, but they also smile, laugh, and joke. When doing the drills, adhere to scientific principles and make sure the drills are safe, challenging, individualized, periodized, and sport-specific. Also check to see that technique and explosiveness are controlled. But, just as important, have a good time. This component of hockey preparation can be as much fun as you want. My favorite quickness and agility drill is tag, either dry-land or on-ice (see page 132). This is a fun drill that is playful and yet very competitive, intense, and highly effective for quickness and agility.

OFF-ICE QUICKNESS AND AGILITY DRILLS

Quickness drills are great for coaches with a large group of athletes. Because most of these drills need little or no equipment, you can work many athletes at once. For 24 athletes, divide them into 6 groups of 4, so while 4 players are completing the drill, 20 are resting. Players rotate in and out of the drills for a 1:5 work-to-relief ratio.

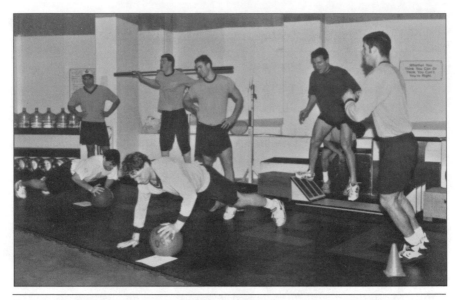

At one end of the Canucks conditioning room, players go through an off-ice practice, altering work and rest intervals.

You can also divide a large group in half so players can work with partners. Partners can be useful for counting the number of foot contacts or for adding a competitive factor to the drills. Coaches can use recovery time to explain the next drill, correct technique, drink fluids, or just as an informal relief phase for players to rest and talk.

Try combining quickness drills with exercises for strength, power, or flexibility. These circuits can be designed so players are partnered and complete the circuit 1:1. While one partner is active, the other rests, and they continually rotate, with no additional rest time.

By factoring in alternating between body parts, and also positioning abdominal exercises, flexibility, or quick-hand drills, for example, partners can move right through the circuit while still receiving the appropriate rest intervals for their legs prior to doing the next quickness or agility drill.

FORWARD LINE DRILLS

Purpose: To help develop quick feet.

Procedure:

1. For method A, face toward a line on the floor.
2. Stand ready with knees slightly flexed and your weight on the toes.
3. Move through the complete pattern, with two quick touches behind the line followed by one foot touch in front of the line.
4. Next, complete the same pattern, but when planting L_3 and R_6, turn your foot in (inwardly rotate leg from hip).
5. For method B, face away from line and complete the reverse pattern (two quick touches in front of line, one step behind line).

Tips:

- Control the pace by clapping or saying "up" every time a foot should touch in front of the line.
- For progression, complete while skipping.

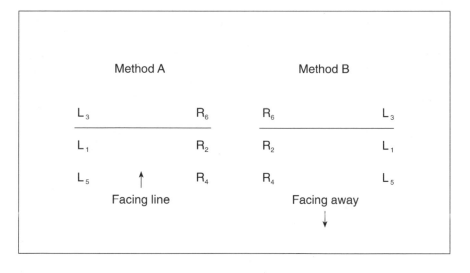

Method A   Method B

L_3 R_6 R_6 L_3

L_1 R_2 R_2 L_1

L_5 ↑ R_4 R_4 L_5

Facing line   Facing away

LATERAL LINE DRILL

Purpose: To help develop quick feet.

Procedure:

1. Start standing to the right of a line on the floor, sideways to the line.

2. Jumping up, touch your right foot and then your left foot to the ground.

3. Cross your outside (right) foot over the inside foot and plant it across the line (R_3).

4. Next, touch your left foot and then right foot, and then cross the left over the right, landing the left across the line (L_6)

5. These are repetitive crossovers back and forth across the line.

6. For method A, keep your foot touches close to the line.

7. For method B, move side to side as wide as possible, so you have more lateral movement. See page 144 for the on-ice version of this drill.

Tip:

- You can control the pace by clapping or saying "cross."

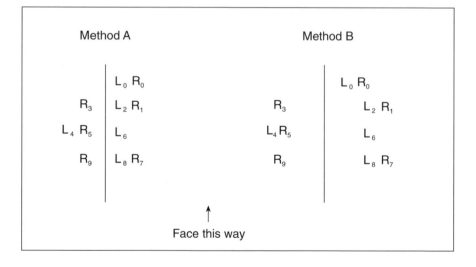

TWO-FOOT LATERAL CONE HOPS

Purpose: To develop quick feet, lateral movement, and stopping speed.

Procedure:

1. Stand beside a cone with feet close together.

2. Hop back and forth sideways over the cone.

3. Land close to the cone and use a low jump height, for a pure quick-feet drill.

4. Also try jumping for more lateral distance, landing as far from the cone as possible.

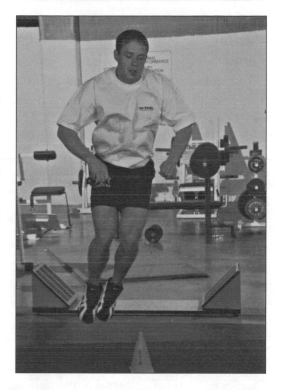

Pavel Bure demonstrates two-foot cone hops. Here he is staying close to the cone while using a low jump height for a quick-feet exercise.

Variations:

A. Stay close to cone, with a low jump height, for a pure quick-feet drill.

B. Jump more for lateral distance, jumping as wide as possible.

C. Stay close to cone, and get good height over cone. Staying close to cone will allow for a quicker directional change after landing.

Tip:

- Count the number of foot contacts within a set time.

THREE-STEP LATERAL BOX JUMPS

Purpose: To help develop quick feet, lateral movement, stopping speed, and agility.

Procedure:

1. Stand behind a stable box, 12 to 15 inches high.

2. Jump up on the box and then immediately explode off to the right side of the box.

3. As soon as your feet touch the floor, try to jump right back up onto the box.

4. Quickly jump off the box and land on the floor behind the box (starting point).

5. Repeat to the left.

6. Continue sequence.

Tip:

- Count the number of foot contacts in a set time.

LATERAL ANGLED BOX JUMPS

Purpose: To develop lateral movement and single-leg power.

Procedure:

1. Push off the left side of angled box with left foot.

2. Land on the right side of angled box with right foot, absorb, and powerfully push over to the left side again.

3. Each time a foot plants on the box, allow enough time for body to move over to that side as well (so there is more knee flexion and position is gained for a longer stride).

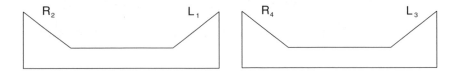

LATERAL ANGLED BOX SHUFFLES

Purpose: To develop quick feet, lateral movement, and agility.

Procedure:

1. Complete the same pattern for lateral angled box jumps but with a quick touch of both feet (one foot at a time) in the middle

2. When contacting angled sides, try to touch upper third of board to work the hip muscles and outside of upper leg.

3. The foot touches in the middle of the board (L_3, R_2, L_5, R_6) should be light and rapid.

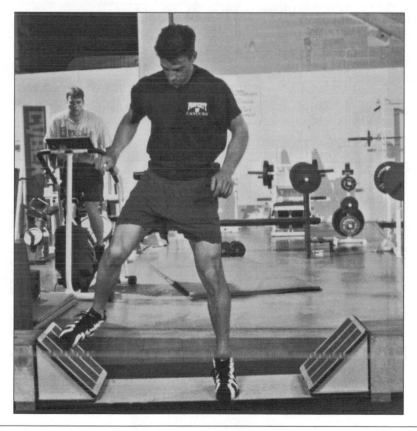

Geoff Courtnall demonstrates the lateral angled box quick-feet shuffles.

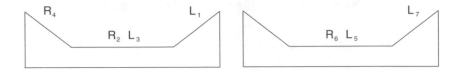

Tip:

- Even when completing low-intensity plyometrics like this one, it is important to have footwear that offers good shock absorption and lateral support. Make sure shoes are laced up tight.

SPLIT-LEG SHUFFLE

Purpose: To help build quick feet and lateral movement muscles.

Procedure:

1. Stand upright with knees slightly flexed, weight on toes, feet close together.

2. Pick up both feet at the same time and land in a wider stance, feet $1\frac{1}{2}$ to 2 feet apart.

3. Quickly pop them back off the floor and land close together, as in the starting position.

4. Continue as rapidly as possible.

Start

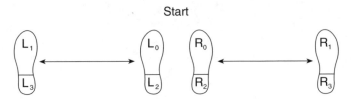

SPLIT-LEG 45-DEGREE SHUFFLES

Purpose: To develop quick feet.

Procedure:

1. Start in the middle of the pattern, feet close together, weight on toes.
2. Pop both feet off the ground, landing left foot forward diagonally and right foot diagonally behind body.
3. Jump back to the starting position.
4. Next jump to a position with right foot forward diagonally and left foot diagonally behind body.
5. Jump back to the starting position.
6. Continue as quickly as possible.

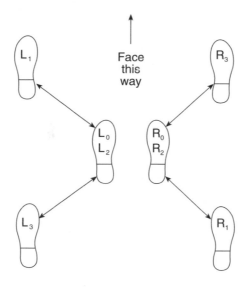

SPLIT-LEG CROSSOVERS

Purpose: To develop quick feet.

Procedure:

1. Start with feet close together, weight on toes.

2. Jump up, moving left foot behind and right foot over top.

3. Land in this position, with legs crossed, then jump up and reverse, left foot moving over the right and right foot moving behind and around.

Tip:

- When first trying this drill, return to the starting stance between each crossover jump.

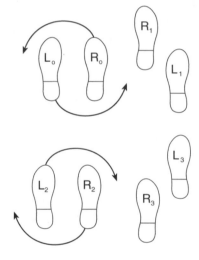

SPEEDTRAXX LATERAL STRIDES

Purpose: To build lateral explosiveness.

Procedure:

1. With one foot on the machine base and hips low, drive off direct laterally with the other foot (see page 96).

2. Use explosive actions, counting the number of reps in a set time.

3. Switch legs and repeat.

TWO-FOOT ANGLED HOPS

Purpose: To help develop quick feet, lateral movement, and directional change.

Procedure:

1. Start with feet close together, weight on toes.
2. Hop forward, jumping at an angle left and right.
3. Reverse direction as quickly as possible, trying to initiate movement in the opposite direction after landing each jump.
4. For method A, hop through with a big angle and not much horizontal distance (width), for more forward quickness.
5. For method B, hop through sharper angles and greater width to emphasize changing direction.

Tip:

- For advanced athletes, try using overspeed tubing, resisted tubing (to build power), or single-leg hops.

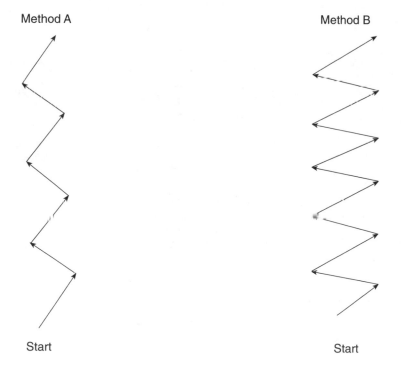

Method A

Start

Method B

Start

LOW-DEPTH JUMPS AND CUT LEFT OR RIGHT

Purpose: To build lateral explosiveness and stopping speed.

Procedure:

1. Start on top of a box, 12 to 15 inches high.

2. Step off box, absorb landing, and react to coach's signal by cutting left or right and sprinting for three or four strides (see photos on this page and the next page).

Tip:

- As improvement is shown, delay the directional signal later and later so that there's less time to read and react.

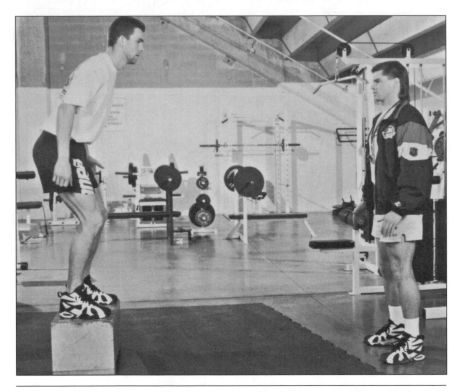

Trevor Linden stands on a short box, prepared for a single rep of low-depth jumps and cut left or right, then executes on the signal after landing (next page).

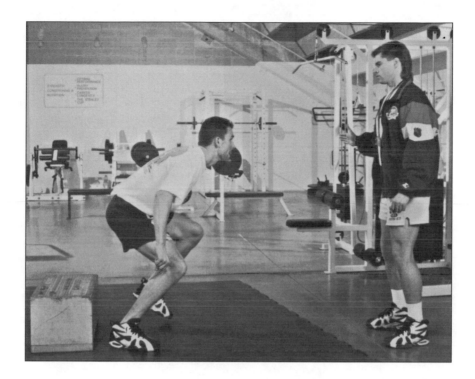

ANKLE TUBING SHADOWING DRILL

Purpose: To develop lateral movement, agility, stopping speed, quick feet, and one-on-one ability.

Procedure:

1. Two players pair up and start by facing each other, knees slightly flexed and weight on their toes.

2. Each player wears a sidewinder tube (a piece of surgical tubing from ankle to ankle that provides resistance to movement).

3. One player is on offense and the other on defense.

4. Players can move only laterally, left to right and right to left.

5. The goal is for the offensive player to "lose" his or her partner, and for the defensive player to stay even with the partner.

6. Start on whistle for a 15-second burst.

OCTAGON DRILL

Purpose: To build quick feet, directional change, and agility.

Procedure:

1. Begin in the middle of the pattern with feet close together, weight on toes, and knees slightly flexed.
2. Hop up to the first position and immediately return to middle.
3. Complete entire pattern without pausing at any position.
4. When landing at each position, overcome the countermovement and spring out to the next spot.
5. Complete once clockwise and once counterclockwise.

Tips:

- Adjust the size of the pattern to each individual's capabilities.
- Advanced athletes can complete with a single leg or while skipping.

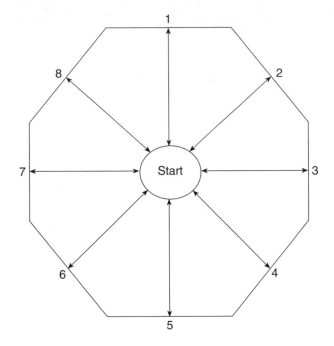

DODGE BALL

Purpose: To develop explosiveness in the hips, abdominals, low back, quadriceps, hamstrings, and gluteals, all important for skating agility. Since explosive movement initiates from the "power center" (hips, abdominals, and low back), dodge ball is also an effective quickness building drill.

Procedure:

1. A player with a tennis ball moves back about 15 feet and tosses the ball right at a partner. Start with easy throws and progressively increase the speed of the throw.

2. The partner moves hips left or right to avoid being hit. He or she should not run away from ball but move hips laterally to avoid being hit.

MEDICINE BALL CHEST PASS (SHORT DISTANCE)

Purpose: Medicine balls are key for explosiveness. If you are trying to move explosively when lifting weights (a bench press, for instance), you have to decelerate near the end of the movement (away from your body) to stop the bar. Only medicine balls allow you to accelerate and explode throughout the entire range of movement.

Procedure: Follow the instructions on page 81, but rather than standing 9 to 12 feet apart, partners stand only 6 feet apart to allow for more rapid-fire passing. This distance depends less on strength and focuses more on pure quickness.

MEDICINE BALL SHOULDER-TO-SHOULDER PASS

Purpose: To build upper-body explosiveness, torso and shoulder power.

Procedure:

1. Complete similar to the medicine ball chest pass, but pass the ball from right shoulder to partner's right shoulder. Then complete a set passing from left to left.

2. When catching the ball, absorb it with trunk rotation and slight knee flexion to develop power in the abdominals and low back.

Tip:

- Advanced athletes can catch and throw the ball with one arm only (i.e., when passing right to right, no catching support with the left hand). This will focus more on the rear shoulder muscles, abdominals, back, and legs to assist the action.

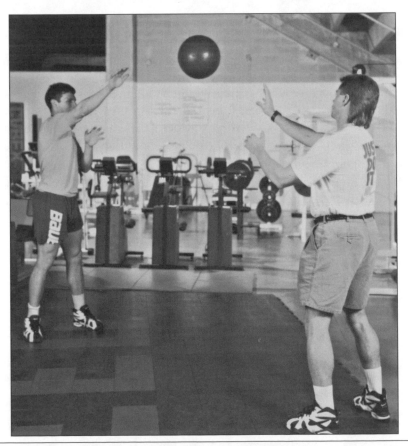

Gino Odjick works on the medicine ball shoulder-to-shoulder pass with trunk rotation.

BACK-TO-BACK PASSES

Purpose: To build rotational power.

Procedure:

1. Stand back to back about 12 inches from a partner.
2. With rapid rotation, pass the ball off one side and rotate over to receive it back on the other side.
3. Complete clockwise and then counterclockwise.

Tip:

- Advanced athletes can rotate farther to meet at the back for a 360-degree pass motion.

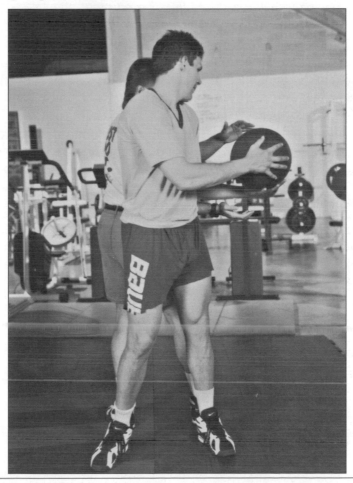

Back-to-back 180-degree passes are shown by Gino Odjick and Pete Twist.

TENNIS BALL DROPS

Purpose: To build quick hands and develop the speed center.

Procedure:

1. Player catching balls starts with knees slightly flexed and hands touching side of quadriceps.
2. Coach stands in front of player and holds up two tennis balls at player's eye level then drops one ball.
3. Player reacts to the dropped ball to catch it before it hits the ground.

Variations:

A: Drop one ball, randomly from left or right hand. Player reacts and catches ball with underhand catch.

B: Player catches the ball with underhand grip, but this time crosses over and catches on the opposite side. That is, if the coach drops the ball out of the right hand, the ball is falling on the player's left side. Player reacts and reaches across to catch ball with right hand.

C: Go through A and B but this time catching the ball with an overhand grip. To get to the ball and cushion the catch (as opposed to quickly slamming the hand down on top of the ball), players will have to use leg and hip quickness to lower themselves rather than trying to go after the ball by throwing down an arm.

Tip:

- Players should quickly drop down using their legs and not bend at the waist to catch the ball. The key is to use the speed center (the hips and upper legs) by quickly dropping the whole body down, keeping the back upright.

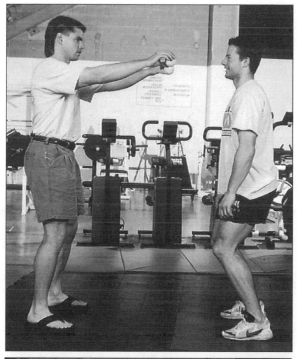

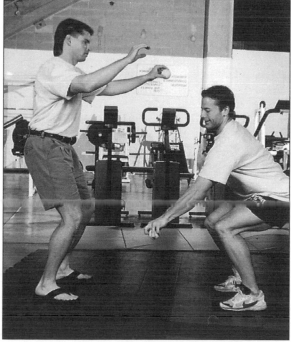

Martin Gelinas shows perfect start and finish form for in-place tennis ball drops.

REACT AND SPRINT TENNIS BALLS DROPS

Purpose: To build first step explosiveness.

Procedure:

1. Coach stands upright holding a tennis ball in each hand. Arms are extended at sides and tennis balls are held about six inches higher than shoulders.

2. Player is positioned a set distance from and facing square to the coach, with slight knee flexion and weight forward on toes, ready to explode into action.

3. Coach drops one ball, and as it leaves the coach's hand, player reacts and sprints after the ball, trying to catch it after only one bounce.

Variations:

A: Same procedure as above but with a sideways start. Player will alternately start facing left or right, having to react, turn, and explode toward dropped ball.

B: Same procedure but player faces *away* from coach (with back to the coach). Player begins in same ready position. Coach calls out "drop" and drops one ball. The player must react, turn with a quick rotation of the hips, sprint out, and cut toward the dropped ball.

Tip:

- This is a great drill for defensemen.

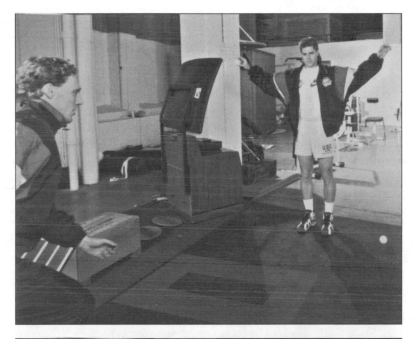

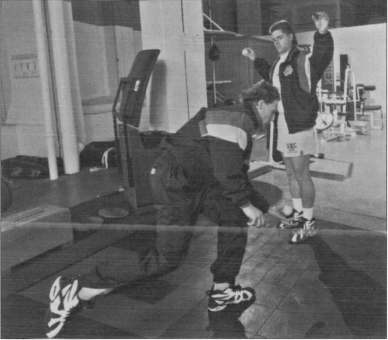

Jyrki Lumme reacts and runs to the ball in this react and sprint tennis ball drop drill.

ON-ICE QUICKNESS AND AGILITY DRILLS

On-ice quickness and agility drills are designed to concentrate first on development of quick feet and agile movements. Then drills can be incorporated which are more sport-specific. Most drills feature puck control, driving to the net or defending the slot area, and utilize quick feet, pivots, crossovers, transition from forward to backward, and many directional changes. You can also integrate segments of your team systems into drills to help transfer agility improvements to team play.

TAG

Purpose: To develop agility, quick feet, reaction abilities. For young players right up through to veteran NHL players, this is my favorite and most effective agility drill.

Procedure:

1. Start with a group of four to six players, who leave their sticks on the bench.

2. One player starts as the "forechecker." All other players hang a small towel from the back of their pants.

3. The forechecker must grab the towel from another player. Once he or she does, then the two of them team up to forecheck the other players.

4. All players with a towel try to evade the forecheckers. As players lose their towels, they become forecheckers.

5. This continues until the last player has lost his or her towel.

6. You don't want players to have an overabundance of open ice. Mark off a boundary so players must face a lot of close one-on-one confrontation.

7. Repeat the drill until each player has had a turn starting as the forechecker.

8. There is no time limit.

OVERSPEED TUBING SIDEWAYS START

Purpose: To develop explosive starts and build agility.

Procedure:

1. Stand sideways to the direction of travel.
2. Coach holds extended tubing.
3. On whistle, cross over, turn, and explode toward the coach.

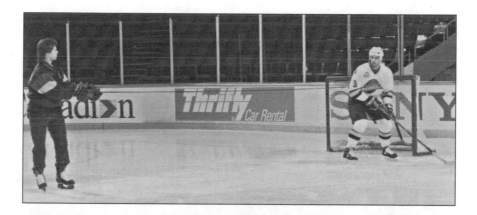

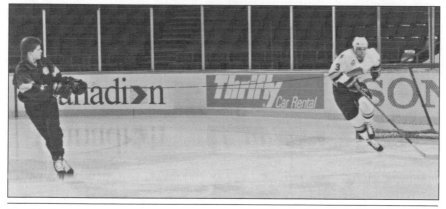

Bret Hedican pushing the limits of explosiveness with the overspeed tubing sideways start with lateral crossovers drill.

RESISTED SPEED/OVERSPEED SKATING

Purpose: To develop quick feet, agility, and direction change.

Procedure:

1. Player begins facing the coach, who is holding the end of the speed tubing.
2. The coach starts moving across ice so the player skates on a diagonal angle.
3. Player skates backward to position 1 through a resisted skate.
4. On whistle, player skates forward overspeed to position 2.
5. When player nears coach and tubing relaxes, player skates backward through a resisted skate to position 3.
6. These movements are repeated across the ice.

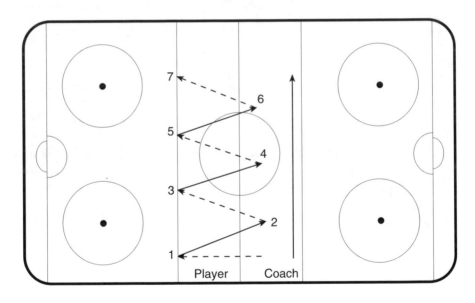

QUICK PIVOT DRILLS I.

Purpose: To build quickness, agility, and first-step acceleration.

Procedure:

1. Always complete carrying a puck.

2. Start on one side of the ice carrying a puck and build up speed to approach the first cone at a high speed.

3. Keep hips low and feet moving fast. Use tight pivots around the cones and pick up feet as soon as you come around cone. Force yourself to pick up your feet sooner than comfortable.

4. Finish with a shot from the slot, and then return to the line.

Tips:

- For advanced skaters, increase the width between cones or decrease the length between cones.

- Players can also go through on a single leg (without a puck), transferring their weight to work off both their inside and outside edges.

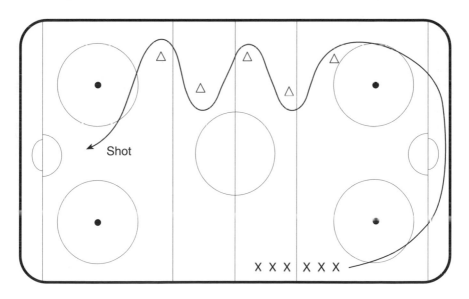

QUICK PIVOT, HIGH DRIVE TO NET

Purpose: To develop quick feet, agility, and puckhandling.

Procedure:

1. Sprint around the net with a puck.

2. Go through cones with tight pivots. Pick up feet and cross over as soon as you come off cone.

3. Drop a short pass to the coach and skate around the last cone.

4. Player will either (1) receive a pass just as coming around the cone, (2) receive a pass breaking through the slot, or (3) tip in a point shot.

5. When players pivot around the last cone, they look for the pass but drive to the net.

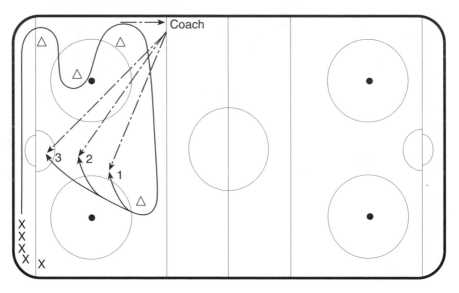

QUICK PIVOT, LOW DRIVE TO NET 2

Purpose: To develop quick feet, agility, and puckhandling.

Procedure:

1. Players start close to the blue line.
2. The coach shoots the puck around boards.
3. Player moves to boards to trap the puck and keep it inside blue line.
4. Player immediately sprints through the cones with quick feet and tight pivots. Force the feet to pick up and cross over coming off the cone.
5. When skating around the cone in the corner, explode and attack the net, moving up and around the slot cone.
6. Shoot as soon as stepping around last cone in the slot.

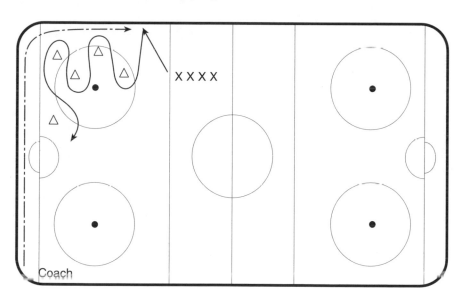

TWO-STEP FORWARD/BACKWARD CIRCLES

Purpose: To build agility and quick feet.

Procedure:

1. Skate around one circle, turning from forward to backward and backward to forward every two steps.

2. Always turn facing inside of circle.

Tips:

-   Use much quicker feet than usual, increasing stride frequency.

-   Initiate direction turn sooner than comfortable, and plant foot and initiate next stride sooner than comfortable.

-   If doing drill properly, player will initially either stumble or be forced out to a wider circle.

-   Keep pressing players to increase foot quickness while also not going too far off circle. They should stay on the circle and force the body to adapt.

-   Encourage earlier foot movement, initiating the first crossover after the player turns backward or forward a lot sooner.

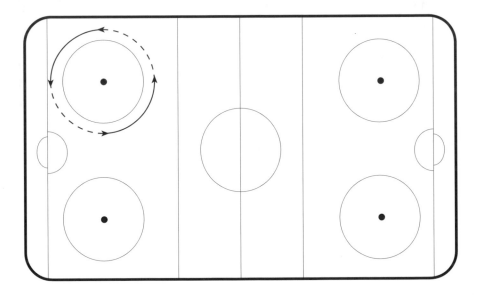

FORWARD/BACKWARD SINGLE TRANSITION

Purpose: To develop agility, direction change, and quick feet.

Procedure:

1. Use two cones or lay a stick on the ice.
2. Move clockwise around stick, turning from forward to backward to forward so you can keep your body square, always facing the same point throughout the drill.
3. Stay as tight to the stick as possible, then work to increase foot speed and speed of movement.
4. Repeat counterclockwise.

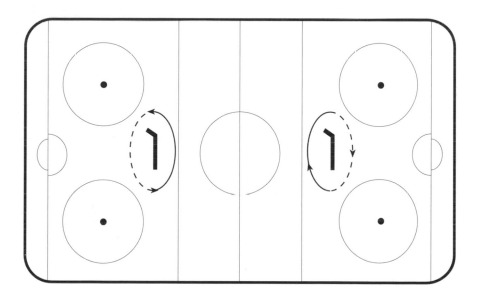

FORWARD/BACKWARD DOUBLE TRANSITION

Purpose: To build agility, direction change, and quick feet.

Procedure: Move forward and backward in and around cones, facing square to end zone throughout pattern.

Tips:

- Position cones as close together as each player can handle.
- Emphasize quick feet, quick transition from forward to backward to forward, and quick shifting of weight.

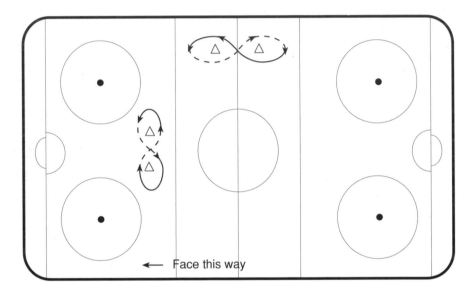

FORWARD/BACKWARD SQUARE BODY FIGURE-8

Purpose: To work on agility and quick feet.

Procedure: Move around figure-8 as quickly as possible, always facing square to end boards.

Tip:

- For advanced athletes, add in passes from the corners or from the top of the slot as the player turns from backward to forward. Time the pass a bit early so the player has to receive the puck just as stepping from backward to forward. Players get a quick shot away while continuing through pattern.

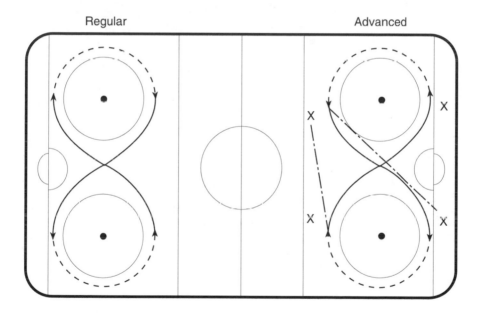

Regular · Advanced

FORWARD/BACKWARD LATERAL CROSSOVER DRILL

Purpose: To build agility and quick feet.

Procedure:

1. Move around pattern as quickly as possible, always facing square to end boards.

2. Skate forward around first circle, turning backward to stay square.

3. Move around circle and cut across slot at hashmarks, turning forward around second circle.

4. Turn backward to finish second circle.

5. As coming off the second circle, use lateral crossovers to move back to starting position.

6. Complete two laps. Rest. Repeat in the opposite direction.

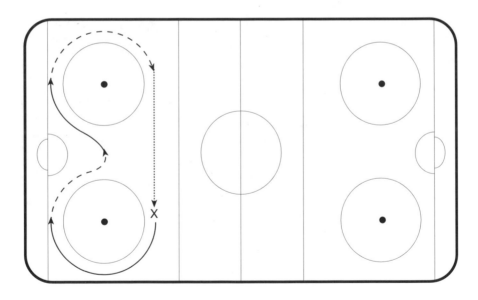

ANKLE TUBING CROSSOVERS

Purpose: To build crossover quickness and power and improve agility.

Procedure:

1. Player wears a Sidewinder (a piece of resistance tubing) connected from ankle to ankle.

2. Player works off of one circle, trying to cross over as quickly as possible.

3. After four sets of 15 seconds (two to the left, two to the right), complete one set to the left and one to the right with no tubing, moving feet as rapidly as possible.

Tip:

- When using resistance tubing, always finish with a natural skating situation so that players can perceive their maximal quickness.

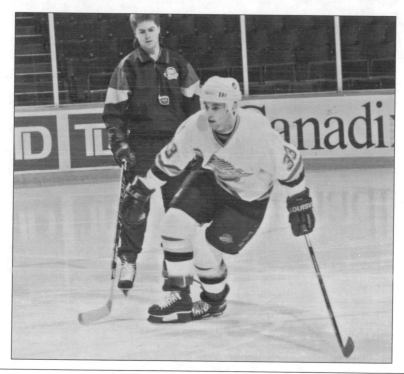

Ankle tubing crossovers demonstrated by Mike Peca.

LATERAL LINE DRILL

Purpose: To build lateral foot speed.

Procedure: Refer to page 114 for drill pattern and instructions. In method A, stay tight to the line, which allows for more rapid footsteps, placing more emphasis solely on foot quickness. In method B of the drill, keep feet close to the ground but move wider for more lateral movement.

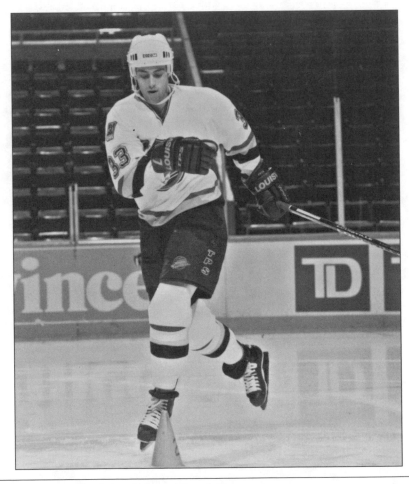

Mike Peca completes a wide lateral line drill.

QUICK-FEET COACH DIRECTIONS 3

Purpose: To build agility, quick feet, and direction change.

Procedure:

1. Player starts on face-off dot.
2. Coach signals left, right, forward, or backward movement.
3. Player moves left or right via crossovers.
4. Signal directional changes in rapid succession.
5. Player reacts, stops, and explodes in next direction.

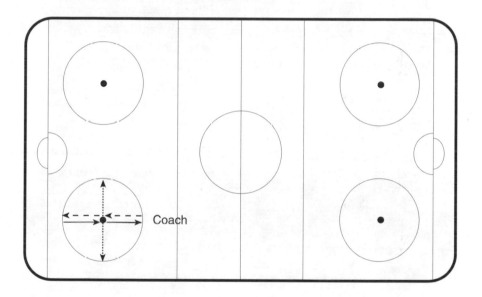

AGILITY STRAP SHADOWING DRILL

Purpose: To develop agility and one-on-one ability.

Procedure:

1. Two players wear a long, lightweight belt with a velcro pad at the end.
2. Players start face to face and connect the two velcro pieces.
3. One player is on defense, the other on offense.
4. The goal for the offensive player is to evade the defensive player and break the velcro connection.
5. The goal for the defensive player is to react and stay with the offensive player so that the belts are not separated.
6. Players can move forward, backward, left, and right, but they cannot spin or turn right around.
7. Use short 15-second bursts.

Tips:

- Pair players of equal ability.
- Mark off a boundary so players must move within a restricted area.

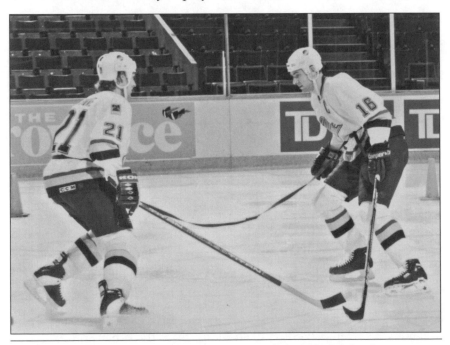

Jyrki Lumme and Trevor Linden challenge each other during the agility strap shadowing drill.

CHAPTER 6

SPEED TRAINING

A coach is making up the day's practice plan. What will be covered at today's practice? The power-play? Three-on-twos? Shooting? Conditioning? Neutral zone transition? These, and many other hockey skills and systems and strategies are taught repeatedly during a season, and all of them are critical to the team's success. But there is one additional component for the practice plan: speed development.

Coaches at all levels teach skating strides, strength development, shooting, bodychecking, and many other skills and parameters that are important to hockey. But many never teach *speed*, although it's recognized as one of the most important components of hockey.

Full-out speed is evident during aggressive forechecking and breakaways. Defensively, backchecking from the other end of the ice back to your net requires speed. While quickness was described as the first gear, speed is the second, third, fourth, and fifth gears. After your first two or three strides, you want to continue accelerating rapidly, attain your top speed as soon as possible, get to as fast a top speed as you can, and then maintain that top speed for as long as you can.

Some athletes are naturally faster than others, just as some are naturally better skaters. But speed development is possible for *all* hockey players. Your players may not progress to being the fastest skaters in the world, but if they become even 10 percent faster, you'll see an incredible difference in the way they perform.

Randy Smythe, president of SpeedCity, Inc. and consultant to pro and college teams, quantifies the incredible potential of speed development: "Increase running stride the length of a penny, and 40-yard dash time for football will decrease 2/10ths of a second. One-hundred meter dash time in track would be down 1/2 second. Add on an increase in stride frequency, and the athlete will run faster still."

Have players simply skate around one face-off circle. Then ask them to skate around the circle faster, and faster. As speed progresses, the players will not be able to stay on the circle, or they'll stumble and fall. They will not have the strength and power around the knees and hips to stay low with bent knees to handle the forces generated at the upper limits of speed.

Most players can develop good skating technique at slow and moderate speeds. But to progress to the upper limits of speed, to full-out speed, and to handle sharp turns at high speeds, the player cannot execute efficient technique without first developing many other physical parameters. There are 10 components that build a base for optimal speed performance. Table 6.1 lists the requisites to high-speed skating.

We can all list past players who were gifted with natural speed. We remember them well because they were exciting to watch. They were blessed with a high capacity for speed, and while they may have worked hard in practices, the majority did not train specifically for speed or even condition the 10 basic components. Imagine the speed these players could have attained if they had developed all 10 components, plus trained for speed improvements! How fast could they have been, and how much longer could they have played? Fortunately, today you have the answers to these questions more within your control.

CONDITIONING FOR SPEED

Improving speed means improving skating technique, including body position, maximizing the use of the skates' edges, staying low with a deep knee-bend, stride power, stride length, and stride frequency. Such

Table 6.1   Ten Requisites to High-Speed Skating

Component	Importance to speed
1. Technique	Critical to skating efficiency.
2. Strength	To fight through hooks and checks and continue striding.
	To support the body in a deep knee position to provide a longer stride so you can apply force over a greater distance each stride.
	To handle high-speed cornering, you need the strength to stay deep with bent knees. Without this strength you will either fall, have to slow down, or take a wider turn.
3. Power	To push off for each stride and power through a long, full stride.
	The power to fight through opponents.
	Selective hypertrophy of fast-twitch muscle fibers.
4. Quickness	For stride frequency.
5. Agility	To suddenly change direction to evade an opponent and continue skating.
6. Flexibility	For stride length and technique.
	For fluidity and range of motion.
7. Anaerobic energy supply	To fuel short bursts of high-intensity muscle action and to delay the fatigue that impedes good technique.
8. Aerobic energy supply	To recover quicker between sprinting situations for more high-speed activity.
9. Body composition	Low body fat facilitates relative strength and efficient movement.
10. Neuromuscular	To increase your ability to activate muscles at a very high rate.

technique relies on strength at the low back, abdominals, hips, knees, and ankles.

A common misconception I've heard from hundreds of coaches, players, and fans is that strength and muscle mass detracts from speed—a big, strong player is muscle bound and slow. This could not be further from the truth. Size, muscle mass, and strength do not make a player slow. With specific training, these factors *contribute* to speed. Shawn Antoski was one of the fastest players I've ever coached, and he was the biggest player on the team and the second strongest. He used his muscle mass and strength for a powerful pushoff on each stride. On today's

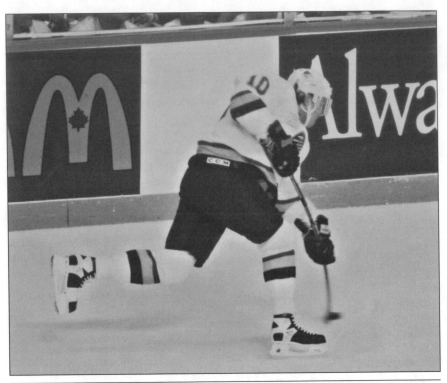

Combining quickness and speed, Pavel Bure unleashes an explosive slapshot.

team, Bret Hedican is the strongest player—and he's now the fastest skater as well.

Which muscles need to be strengthened to build a base for speed? Developing the quadriceps (thigh), calf muscles, and hip extensors provides a powerful forward stride. Working the hamstrings (back of the upper leg) and hip flexors gives you the strength to pull your leg back in and position it for another pushoff. Training the lower back muscles and abdominals aids all parts of the stride, and also benefits turning and lateral movement. Strengthening the adductor and abductor muscles improves lateral movement and plays a key role in both forward and backward skating. Developing the arm and shoulder muscles is also necessary, as these muscles are very active during all acceleration and high-speed skating. What it comes down to is that you need a strength base in *all* major muscle groups before you can safely begin training for speed. And you need to continually improve your strength to make further speed progressions.

The exercises and drills in this chapter develop stride length, stride power, stride frequency, and muscle contractile speed. Your goal is to *lengthen a stride* so that you're applying force over a greater distance.

Player A takes 12 skating strides for one length of the ice. Player B takes 16 strides and longer time. Player A is able to apply force over a greater distance every stride, getting more distance from each stride.

A *more powerful stride* also contributes to speed. Player A can take 10 strides. Player B also takes 10 strides that are equal in length and frequency. But player A has a more powerful stride and gets a stronger pushoff, getting greater drive from each stride and thus covering more distance in the same amount of time. This is what players do to increase speed—they take long strides with a strong pushoff to build and maintain speed.

Stride frequency takes speed to another level, contributing by quickly pulling the leg back in and planting the skate as rapidly as possible so you're positioned to push off again. Stride frequency involves how fast you can pick up your trail leg, pull it back in, and put it down to ready for the next pushoff. For many players, stride frequency is an underdeveloped area that can really improve speed capabilities.

The goal of speed training is to produce as much force as you can in as short a time as you can—*contractile speed* contributes to this. Speed development drills are done full-out. It is high-velocity conditioning. The main types of activities used to develop speed are resistive and overspeed exercises, explosive strength training, and plyometrics.

Resisted Speed Exercises

To develop stride power and improve stride length, apply resistance to force the athlete to work harder and overcome the resistance. Resisted speed exercises and drills use partners, tubing, straps, weighted vests, speed chutes, and running uphill and upstairs to help improve leg drive. On the ice, resisted speed drills help players maintain a positive angle from the hip to the ice, get the best leg drive, and use the skates' edges to generate maximum force.

Overspeed Exercises

Overspeed exercises and drills key on stride frequency and contractile speed. They force players to run or skate much faster than they're accustomed to. The brain must signal the muscles to fire much quicker.

In these drills, players are pulled or run downhill, forcing them to increase stride frequency to move the foot forward and plant it in time for the next stride. These exercises help show players the speed they're really capable of. They realize they have the potential to move that fast. When this occurs, the neuromuscular system learns to fire the muscles faster and adapts to a higher level of speed capacity.

Chris Chelios

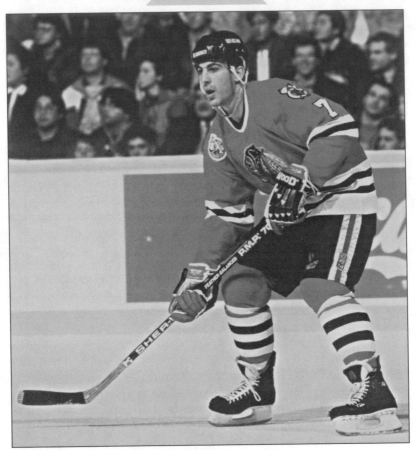

"Compared to 10 years ago, today's players are in top condition. Players are bigger and faster because of their work ethic and their conditioning," says Chris Chelios, winner of the Norris Trophy as the NHL's best defenseman in 1989, 1993, and 1996. "There's only so much you can do on the ice. I think off-ice conditioning is the key. Most of my conditioning drills are for the legs. That's the most important component—to get your legs in the best condition you possibly can. Top players are in such good shape that if you don't work hard on your leg conditioning, you won't be able to keep up," stresses Chelios. "The season is so long and grueling, I can't emphasize enough your physical preparation."

Chelios has skated for 13 years in the NHL and has appeared in seven NHL All-Star games. He has also competed for the U.S. National Team, the U.S. Olympic Team, and Team USA in the 1991 Canada Cup. From this experience, Chelios recommends, "You have to train properly and professionally. You need really good coaches, because sometimes you can exercise and actually hurt your body or develop counterproductive to hockey. You need the right type of coaching to make sure you condition specifically for hockey."

SPEED TRAINING GUIDELINES

To get the most out of the time you spend on speed development, follow these guidelines:

1. First build a strength base, increase lean muscle mass, and develop the energy systems (for supply and recovery). Players risk injury if they take on high-intensity speed training without these base parameters. In general, players should be able to squat their body weight and have a good level of athleticism before taking on speed training. High-intensity speed exercises (e.g., jumping heights over 15 inches or hopping for distance) require a solid base of strength in the legs and torso.

2. Use a low volume of work initially, keeping intensity low. Low intensity includes using moderate speeds and, if using plyometrics, low jumping heights. Then progress to high-speed movements, but still keep plyometric intensity low. Complete plyometrics at top speed, but do not go overboard with the heights of jumps and the heights of benches. Instead, emphasize speed and increased lateral or linear horizontal jump and hop distances. Depth jumps and other plyometrics from high heights pose an injury risk. Since players rarely jump from two- or three-foot heights during a hockey game, keep jumping and bounding heights low to moderate!

3. Players should have good form and proper technique. You don't want to practice completing incorrect movements faster. Assess balance, foot placement, ready positions, edges, absorption, and use of arms during acceleration.

4. Break in to speed development with a low volume and low frequency.

5. Emphasize quality over quantity. Don't confuse the most physically exhausting workout with the best workout. Some physiological

parameters are best developed by physically overloading the body. But speed is best improved with bursts of high-intensity movement, interspersed with active rest and recovery. You are teaching your body to move fast, not slow and fatigued—rest enough between repetitions so you don't impede technique.

6. Once speed is improved on-ice, start carrying a puck through each speed and overspeed drill. But don't sacrifice speed for puck control; players likely already know how to carry the puck going a slow to moderate speed. Maintain top speed and learn to handle the puck at these speeds.

7. Keep speed development drills between 5 and 15 seconds—long enough to allow players to draw on their anaerobic energy systems for full-out efforts but not so long that fatigue affects their speed. Some hockey books list anaerobic glycolysis drills, such as stop-and-start line drills, for developing speed. But if you compare a player's skating technique for the first and last 10 seconds of these drills, you'll see that technique becomes terribly flawed as players get tired. Such exercises just rehearse skating slowly with poor technique. They do build leg endurance, but they don't increase upper end speed. Additionally, 15 seconds is also a practical speed limit, since players can skate one full lap of the ice in that time—they would never skate longer in a game without having to decelerate, stop, or change direction.

8. Allow approximately a minute of relief between drills. As the practice progresses, rely on feedback from the players on how they feel—are they still fatigued, or are they ready to go? Insufficient rest intervals leaves the players prefatigued at the start of the next drill. This results in a less powerful pushoff, shorter strides, less knee-bend, and a slower stride rate. To improve speed capabilities, players need to produce a more powerful pushoff through a longer stride, deep knee flexion, and a greater leg turnover.

9. Coaches must encourage players to challenge themselves. If I'm coaching a player on the ice, and he doesn't stumble or fall now and then, I know he's not challenging his capabilities. If you let them, most players will keep within a comfortable limit that they are already confident they can execute well. If my player is pushing himself to another level, if he is extending himself to try to complete drills and skills with greater speed than he is accustomed to, he is initially bound to stumble or lose control of the puck. Once he practices this faster speed, he'll eventually be able to skate at this level flawlessly. Encourage and reward short-term failure so players will extend themselves past their proficiency limits to produce long-term improvement. There's nothing more admirable than a willingness to learn and improve.

10. During the preseason, I use up to 30 to 40 speed drill sets; during the season I may have 10 speed drill sets for players before the regular team practice.

OFF-ICE SPEED DRILLS AND EXERCISES

HANG TIME BOUNDING

Purpose: To improve stride length and stride power.

Procedure:

1. From a stationary start, push off with one foot to move your body in a straight line.

2. Land on the opposite leg, absorbing the landing and immediately pushing off to continue bounding, alternating from left to right leg.

3. Use long and powerful strides to get as much vertical height and linear distance as possible each stride.

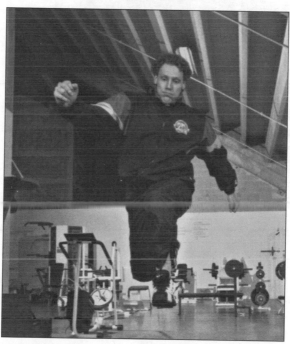

Jyrki Lumme gets great height and distance on his hang time bounding, trying to "hang" in the air as long as possible.

LATERAL BOUNDING

Purpose: To build stride length and stride power.

Procedure:

1. Push off one foot at a 45-degree angle, jumping as high and traveling as far as possible.

2. Land on one leg, absorb the landing, and push off to travel the opposite direction.

3. Jump from left to right to left, down the floor at 45-degree angles.

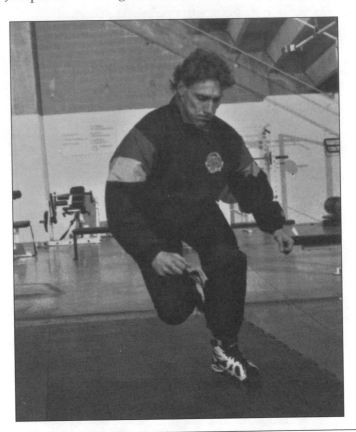

Jyrki Lumme strides out at a 45-degree angle, absorbs the landing, and strides out the opposite direction during these lateral bounding movements.

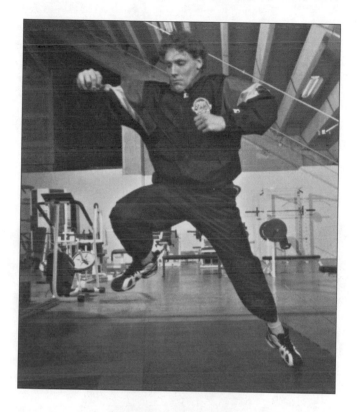

SPEED SQUATS

Purpose: To increase stride power and contractile speed.

Procedure:

1. Perform a standard squat technique (see page 87-88), moving through each rep explosively.

2. Lower into the squat as fast as you can, and immediately drive back up, trying to minimize the pause at the bottom. Extend legs as fast as you can.

3. Continue through the entire set.

Tip:

• Use from low (zero or an empty Olympic bar) to moderate weight loading.

JUMP SQUATS

Purpose: To build stride power and contractile speed.

Procedure:

1. Lower into a squat position and rise back up, powerfully extending legs right through to a jump position. Drive up powerfully enough to bring feet right off the ground.
2. As soon as the feet touch the ground, lower into a squat.
3. At the bottom, try to minimize any pause and drive back up into another jump.
4. Continue through the set.

Tips:

- Be sure to use perfect squat technique for protection against injury.
- Use a light (zero to empty Olympic bar) weight loading.

LUNGE JUMPS

Purpose: To build leg and hip power, stride length, hip flexibility, and contractile speed.

Procedure:

1. Stand upright with feet shoulder-width apart.
2. Step out with left leg and lower into a lunge position, with left knee at a 90-degree angle, left quadricep parallel to the floor, left knee over left foot (but not past toes), and hips as low to the ground as possible. Right leg extends behind body.
3. From that starting position, jump up in place and switch leg positions midair, so that upon landing, the right leg is lunged out in front and the left leg extends behind the body.
4. Absorb landing and jump right back up, switching legs to land in starting position.
5. Continue sequence.

Tip:

- Use a light weight loading (zero to empty Olympic bar).

SPEEDTRAXX LINEAR STRIDING

Purpose: To build leg and hip power and contractile speed.

Procedure:

1. Position both tracks straight back in a linear direction.
2. Place toes on tracks, hips low, grasp handles, and support chest on chest pad.
3. Extend right leg to push track back as far as possible
4. While moving into knee and hip flexion to return your right foot to the starting position, extend left leg to drive the left track back as far as possible.
5. Continue alternating legs with explosive, long strides.

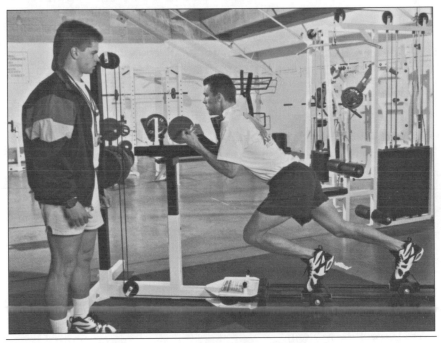

Speedtraxx linear striding is performed by Trevor Linden.

TWO-STEP STAIR SPRINTS

Purpose: To help develop stride power and stride length.

Procedure:

1. Use powerful strides to sprint up a steep set of stairs two steps (or more) at a time.

2. Walk back down slowly, one step at a time, and finish rest interval at bottom.

Tip:

- Also complete reps using a sideways crossover sprint. Turn 90 degrees so left shoulder is pointed up the stairs and right shoulder down the stairs. Keeping the body square, cross your right over the left to sprint up the stairs. Repeat facing the opposite direction to cross left over right. This also helps hip flexibility.

LATERAL BENCH SQUATS

Purpose: To build leg power.

Procedure:

1. Start with left leg flexed and left foot supported up on a bench, hips off to the right side, and right foot planted on the floor two to three feet from the bench.

2. Quickly extend both legs to jump up and to the left, so you can land with right foot on the bench and left foot two to three feet to the left of the bench. Flex both knees and lower hips.

3. Immediately jump back up and laterally to the right.

4. Continue alternating sides through set.

Tips:

- Keep back upright.

- Begin this drill with no weight. Progress to only an empty Olympic bar. Emphasize speed of movement versus increasing resistance.

STRIDE LENGTH MATCH RUNNING

Purpose: To increase stride length.

Procedure:

1. Team a tall and short player together.
2. The tall player runs at about 80 percent speed, and the short player tries to match the tall player's length of stride.

Tip:

- For this and the following matching drill, If you do not have a partner, or as a way to quantify and monitor progression, you can complete the drills individually by marking the desired foot placements with tape or cones on the ground.

STRIDE FREQUENCY MATCH RUNNING

Purpose: To increase stride frequency.

Procedure:

1. A tall and short player are partners.
2. The short player runs at 90 percent speed, while the tall player tries to match the short player's stride frequency, planting his or her foot at the same time as the short player does, step for step.

DOWNHILL OVERSPEED RUNNING

Purpose: To increase stride frequency and contractile speed.

Procedure:

1. This involves sprinting down a hill that has a 3 to 7 percent grade.
2. Sprint for up to 15 seconds before braking to slow down.
3. Walk back to the starting position.

Tip:

- If the decline is too great and stride frequency increased too much for a player's ability, he or she will begin landing on the heels instead of the balls of the feet. This is actually a braking action to help slow down and control the body's movement, which eliminates any potential speed benefits.

ON-ICE SPEED DRILLS AND EXERCISES

FULL-SPEED SPRINT WITH SKATING START

Purpose: To increase stride frequency, stride power, stride length, and contractile speed.

Procedure:

1. Skate straight down one side of ice at 80 percent speed.
2. Build up to 90 percent speed around end with quick crossovers.
3. Come out of corner wide and accelerate to 100 percent speed at face-off hashmarks.
4. Sprint full-out straight down to far face-off hashmarks.
5. Recover in middle of ice.

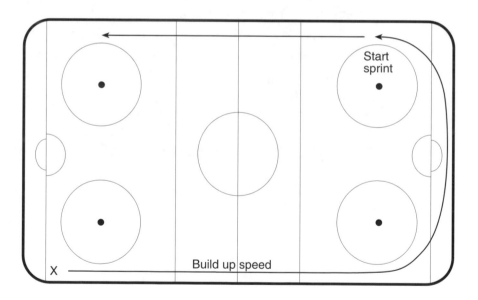

FLOW SPEED DRILL

Purpose: To develop high-speed skating and puck control.

Procedure:

1. Start one at a time.

2. Accelerate around net and sprint through pattern, staying wide to maximize speed.

3. Stay low with deep knee-bend to take face-off dot turn at a high speed.

4. Accelerate around center face-off circle and receive a pass at full speed.

5. Finish by driving to the net for a shot.

6. Next one in line starts as the player ahead pivots around blue line face-off dot (the one closest to line-up).

Tips:

- For high-speed puck control, players can leave with a puck, carry the puck through the drill, passing once to the coach after players turn around face-off dot, and receive the pass back as they approach the final blue line.

- Advanced players can leave with a puck and complete as many give-and-goes as possible, yet not at the expense of skating speed.

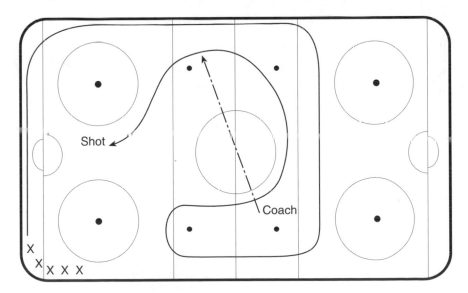

PARTNER FLOW SPEED RACE

Purpose: To help develop high-speed skating.

Procedure:

1. Two players leave at same time on whistle.

2. When skating around pattern, players have to stay *outside* of circles.

3. The first player to cross the center red line (at right of circle) receives a pass and finishes with shot from top of slot.

4. Trailing player skates wide around face-off circle and drives to net for rebound.

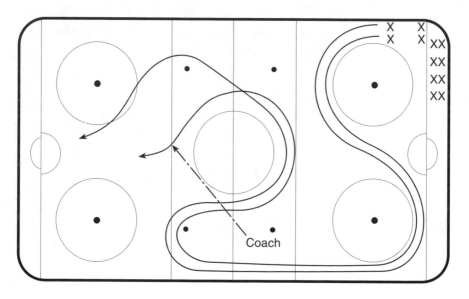

PARTNER FLOW PUCK RACE

Purpose: To develop high-speed skating and acceleration.

Procedure:

1. Two players start at diagonally opposite face-off circles, stationary on the face-off dot.

2. On the whistle, they sprint out to face-off dot 1, around 2, over to 3, back down to the starting position (4), and off to center, racing for the one puck sitting on the center face-off dot.

3. At center, players must cross their right hand side of the puck to avoid collision.

4. Player who reaches puck first continues on for a shot in the net.

5. Player losing race can opt to turn backward and defend net one-on-one, but avoids head-on checking.

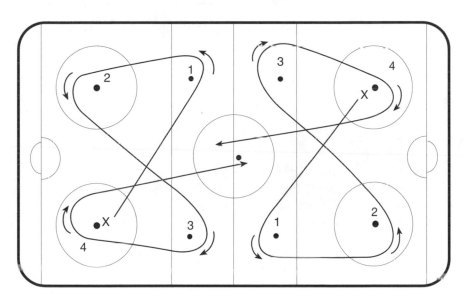

SPEED CHANGE-UP DRILL

Purpose: To develop acceleration ability and stride frequency.

Procedure:

1. Skate at 80 percent speed around ice.
2. On whistle, quickly accelerate to full speed, and maintain top speed.
3. On next whistle, decelerate back to 80 percent speed.
4. Vary the time between whistles, blowing the whistle every 1 to 5 seconds, so players practice reacting and quickly shifting gears.
5. Continue for up to 20 seconds before players skate easy for a rest interval.

OVERSPEED TUBING FORWARD

Purpose: To increase stride frequency, acceleration, and contractile speed.

Procedure:

1. Player wearing overspeed tubing stands ready to accelerate with knees flexed and hips low.
2. Coach pulls tubing to a stretched position.
3. On whistle, player accelerates straight forward.
4. Coach should also move in the same direction, to help keep a stretch on the tubing and lengthen the time the player remains in an overspeed environment.

Tips:

- Players should be well warmed up before attempting this drill.
- This is a great drill to end practice with, so players leave last remembering the feeling of their body and feet moving at this speed.
- Try matching one of your fastest skates with one of your slowest skaters. From a skating start, have the faster skater take off around the ice wearing one end of the tubing, the slower skater wearing the other end of the tubing and trying to meet the speed. Monitor the degree of stretch on the tubing and whistle down drill if degree of stretch becomes unsafe.

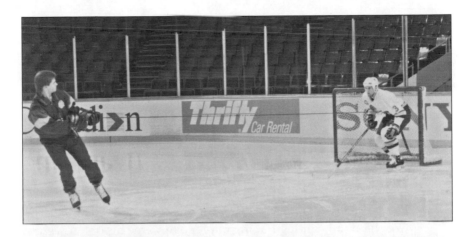

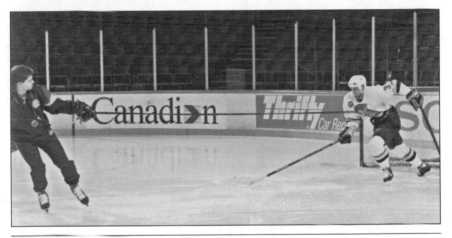

Coach Twist helps Bret Hedican work on his acceleration and stride frequency, forcing a greater rate of leg turnover with an overspeed tubing drill.

OVERSPEED TUBING BACKWARD

Purpose: To build skating speed.

Procedure:

1. Set-up is similar to overspeed tubing forward, but backward can be better accomplished with a dynamic start.

2. With the player wearing the tubing already skating backward, the coach will hold end of tubing and skate forward, leading the player, keeping a slight stretch on the tubing.

3. Maintain this position around the ice, forcing high-speed cross-overs around the ends of the ice.

RESISTED LATERAL CROSSOVERS

Purpose: To increase stride power and stride length.

Procedure:

1. Player starts sideways to coach, wearing a resistance belt or harness.
2. Coach holds end of belt and skates pointed directly toward player.
3. Player starts on whistle, moving laterally by crossing over and pushing off.
4. Coach initially glides, having player overcome his or her weight as resistance.
5. After the player develops momentum, the coach can point toes in or drag one skate behind to slightly increase resistance.
6. Repeat, crossing over opposite side.

Tips:

- You'll notice that players more readily adopt a longer stride to enhance the power and the pushoff phase to help overcome the resistance.
- Make sure the player generates a strong pushoff from both the outside and inside crossover foot.
- Position the belt behind the player's arm, so it does not inhibit skating mechanics.

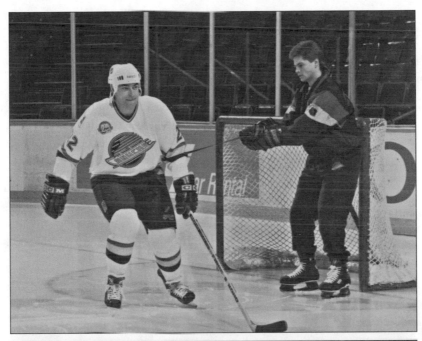

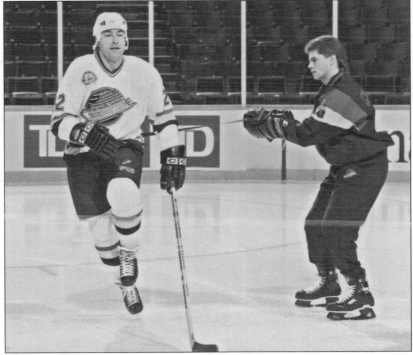

Resisted lateral crossovers help Jeff Brown develop strength for lateral movement and directional changes during one-on-ones.

FORWARD/BACKWARD RESISTED SKATING

Purpose: To increase stride power and stride length.

Procedure:

1. Player begins from a stationary position, positioned to either accelerate forward or backward.
2. Coach holds resistance belt or harness.
3. On whistle, player accelerates while coach glides behind.
4. Once player develops momentum, coach increases resistance by using skate edges.

Tip:

- Encourage long, powerful strides.

LET-GOES

Purpose: To build stride power, stride length, and acceleration.

Procedure:

1. On whistle, skate full-out with powerful strides under a resisted condition.
2. After five or six strides, coach lets go of resistance and yells "go," giving players a strong jump and allowing an accelerated rate of leg turnover.

Tip:

- Players begin with full-out, powerful strides, but they must also be encouraged to kick in a second effort upon hearing "go!" to maximize their acceleration at the let-go phase.

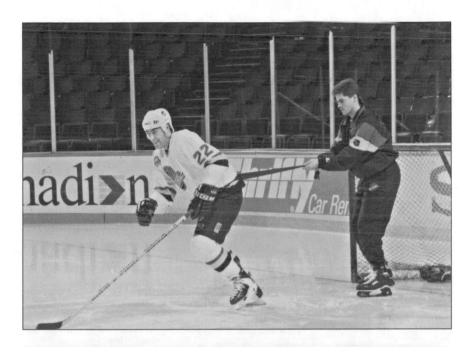

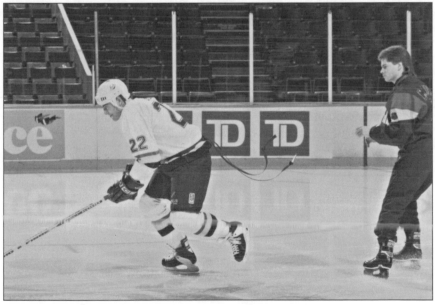

Let-goes start with a resisted condition, with the player accelerating with powerful strides. At some point before leg fatigue sets in, the coach drops the belt while yelling "go!" At the let-go stage, Jeff Brown increases his acceleration.

RESISTED/OVERSPEED POWER PIVOTS

Purpose: To build stride power, stride frequency, and contractile speed.

Procedure:

1. Position cones so player will skate down ice from side to side, around each cone.

2. For the resisted condition, the coach holds the end of the resistance harness and glides down the middle of cones, while the player powers around each cone.

3. For the overspeed condition, the coach leads the player, skating down the middle of the cones to maintain a slight stretch on the overspeed tubing.

4. Player must move around cone and pick feet up right away to meet the demands of the overspeed condition.

Tip:

- During overspeed, having the coach stay down the middle of the cones will place the player's emphasis on moving quickly around each cone and coming off each cone with quick strides.

CHAPTER 7

NUTRITION FOR HOCKEY PERFORMANCE

Your body has over one billion moving parts and 600,000 miles of veins and arteries, and if you took your lungs out of your body, opened them up, and laid them cell-by-cell on the ground (caution: do not try this at home), they would cover an area bigger than an Olympic ice surface. Your body is such an intricate machine—the only machine in the world that is not fully understood by anyone. In comparison, an automobile is a very simple machine, but people know that using anything but the proper fuel makes a car run poorly or break down altogether. Consequently, people would never think of putting anything but gasoline in their cars. But people don't have the same concern for their own bodies—they try to keep them running using all kinds of wrong fuel. The result is a body that sputters and eventually breaks down! From a functional point of view, the typical North American is 30 years older physiologically than his or her chronological age indicates. For example, an active 60-year-old with a healthy diet has a similar physical capacity to a sedentary 30-year-old with a poor diet.

Science has proven again and again that a well-balanced diet promotes good health. Besides nutrition's immediate benefits to an athlete for hockey performance, refining eating habits is very important for present and long-term health. A high-fat, low-nutrient diet is a risk factor for many illnesses—from susceptibility to colds and flus to major diseases. There are life-giving and life-taking foods. Low fitness and poor nutrition can help cause osteoporosis, broken bones, headaches, constipation, allergies, skin irritations, kidney stones, gall stones, gout, obesity, high blood pressure, diabetes, heart disease, strokes, stomach cancer, pancreatic cancer, prostate cancer, breast cancer, colon cancer, liver disease, and autoimmunity disorders. The good news is that we can choose not to fuel these maladies through our diets and habits—both food selection and activity level are completely within our control.

It is within our control, and it is up to *you*, because society does not yet embrace a preventative philosophy. The medical community still supports a reactionary approach, teaching doctors to prescribe drugs to "treat" ailments. In North America, there isn't really even a healthcare system—it is actually a disease treatment system. But no doctor or pharmaceutical company has ever been able to replace nutrition and exercise as the best prescription for promoting health and longevity.

Many physicians, for example, believe that an elevated blood pressure is a natural concomitant of the aging process, and they prescribe antihypertensive medications for elevated blood pressure. But blood pressure remains *normal* with increasing age when accompanied by a regular fitness program. Similarly, most medical plans will pay for a $50,000 heart bypass surgery but will not pay for a $90 consultation with a nutritionist to receive information that can prevent the need for a heart bypass. Medicine may treat the symptoms, but only you personally can treat the cause. It is permanent lifestyle changes that can prevent many illnesses and debilitating states, and while surgery or drugs may help extend one's life, it is exercise and nutrition that will keep you fully functional and healthy longer into life—the idea being not just to add years to your life, but life to your years.

The great news is that if you eat for hockey success, you'll also take care of your health. Aspiring athletes will buy into optimal nutrition to help them achieve their hockey goals. Hockey may be the reason, excellence the motivation, involvement in the game the gratification, and hockey success the immediate reward, but long-term health and wellness is the ultimate benefit.

Don Cherry

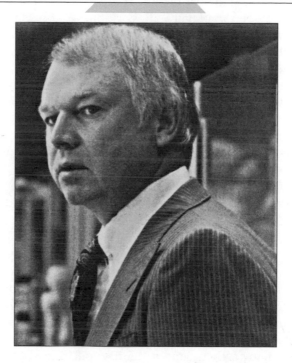

Don Cherry's Boston Bruins had a reputation as a hard-working team that was physically better prepared than the opposition. He seemed to have a knack for getting a lot more on-ice success out of a team that on paper did not seem as capable. Coach Cherry used many psychological strategies on both his players and their opponents, while also fostering cohesion within the team. He attributes his teams' successes to being in the best "game shape" of any team. "You should have seen some of the Montreal Canadiens' practice scrimmages back in the 60s and 70s. It was unbelievable. I learned from watching Toe Blake. All of his scrimmages were high tempo. They needed to do this to prepare them to go all-out in games. I carried that into the Boston Bruins. I wouldn't have long practices, because players learn to pace themselves. We would only practice for an hour or so, but it was full tilt. Everything was quick, done in short bursts. And no standing around. Sometimes coaches start practice, and then take a long time explaining drills or systems, and the players are cold again. Keep them moving."

"Coaches should try and keep it fun. Even in the NHL you can see some teams having fun in practice. There's no doubt in my mind—a 35-year-old veteran player will work harder if he's having fun. Obviously, the younger the player, the more important this becomes. But the fun aspect has to be built into game-specific practices. I never did things in practice that never happened in a game. Every drill we did was in game conditions, and everything was in short bursts, because hockey is played in short bursts. Shifts are 30 seconds or so. That's all they are. We were the best conditioned team in any sport. We used to outwork every team we met. There had to be a mental willingness to do that, but conditioning allowed us to do it."

"The Bruins were in the best shape. That helped us be successful in the playoffs, and it's why we got a lot out of the talent we had."

For hockey, nutrition is a key link between physical preparation and improved game performance. No matter how hard you work on and off the ice, without optimal nutrition you'll never achieve optimal hockey performance. As you prepare for and recover from a hockey game, there are precise times to put specific foods and fluids into your body.

While most athletes know they need carbohydrates to fuel their sport participation, many of them cannot identify specific carbohydrate foods. Nor can they identify high-fat or high-protein sources. The inability to distinguish between foods makes it difficult for them to eat a balanced diet and consume the right foods at the right times. Even for those with the best knowledge of nutrition, eating an optimal hockey performance diet is a challenge given the schedule of games, practices, off-ice conditioning, travel, and the variety of environments in which they must eat, including buses, planes, hotels, arenas, and restaurants. Many athletes express frustration about trying to eat properly on the road.

In this chapter I'll describe scientifically proven nutrition guidelines that will optimize hockey performance. You'll learn how to delay fatigue, speed postgame recovery, promote prevention of illness, and assist the rehabilitation process after an injury.

A coach who demands hard work from players has the responsibility to teach them what and when to eat in order to fuel the very hard work required of them. And players who are working hard to improve *deserve* to get optimal results from their efforts. Once they realize the power of certain food choices and how they can eat for hockey success, they'll turn to nutrition as a competitive edge. And they'll adopt it more willingly than you might expect because it is an *effortless* edge. Usually improvements in hockey performance require extra physical exercise or practice time. If a player knows that simply choosing food A over food B provides twice the energy on the ice, it will be a natural and easy choice to make.

But sometimes once players have decided to eat right, it's still hard for them to find the proper foods at the proper times. In such cases, coaches need to help set up the opportunities to eat performance-enhancing foods. It is also important for coaches to adopt the same nutrition guidelines they are teaching, especially when they are with their players. If you are preaching hard work, physical preparation, and good nutrition, then just don't preach it—live it!

NUTRIENTS

Six nutrients within four main food groups are essential for health and hockey success. The nutrients are carbohydrates, fat, protein, vitamins, minerals, and water. The food groups are grain products, fruits and vegetables, milk products, and meat and meat alternatives.

Carbohydrates

Carbohydrates are the main source of energy during a hockey game. Complex carbohydrates come from the grain products group (formally known as the breads and cereals group) and the fruits and vegetables group. Simple carbohydrates are foods like table sugar and honey. Both these starches and sugars are stored in the blood, liver, and muscles as glucose and glycogen, available to fuel on-ice activity.

Athletes are encouraged to get 65 percent or more of their daily caloric intake from carbohydrates. (The average North American diet consists of 30 percent carbohydrates.) Most of this should be complex carbohydrates, with no more than 10 percent simple carbohydrates. Carbohydrates for hockey can be classified differently, by glycemic index. This is important to sport performance and will be discussed later in this chapter.

Fat

Fat does have some positive roles for the body: providing energy for submaximal activity and protection for the body during impact, and serving many operational functions such as aiding digestion and vita-min transfer. But too much fat is very unhealthy and makes movement less efficient, because the extra weight of fat does not contribute to movement, as muscles do. Fat comes mainly from "added" sources, the extras we put on our main meal—butter, margarine, mayonnaise, salad dressing—and from baked goods like cakes, pies, cookies, and muffins. Fat is also high in some foods in the meat and meat alternatives group, the milk products group, and various processed foods, fried foods, and what we call "junk food." The average North American diet is made up of 45 percent fat, whereas it should be no more than 25 percent. Elite athletes can lower their fat intake to 20 percent of their daily calories, while young kids can move it up to 30 percent.

Certain fats, called *saturated* fats, can build up in your arteries and cause clogs or blood clots, which can lead to heart attacks or strokes. These fats are solid at room temperature and include butter, margarine, fried foods, meat fat, coconut oil, and palm oil. Cholesterol, another artery-clogger as risky as saturated fat, is found only in animal sources such as meat and dairy products.

Protein

Protein's well-known function is to repair and build muscle tissue. Protein, made up of amino acids, is used as an energy source only if there are not enough carbohydrates available. The average diet intake for protein is 25 percent. Athletes' intakes should be less, about 15 to 20 percent protein. Since most people already consume much more protein than their body can use for muscle growth, athletes do not need to take protein supplements. Excess protein does not make you stronger, and it is *not* stored as muscle—it is usually stored as fat.

The best sources for protein are the meat and meat alternatives and the milk products groups. Since many good protein sources are also high in fat, athletes need to choose their protein sources wisely. Table 7.1 compares the fat content of common protein foods. You can see that split peas, lentils, kidney beans, and skim milk are the "stars" of the protein foods—they are high in protein and carbohydrate and low in fat.

Vitamins and Minerals

Vitamins and minerals are not an energy source, but they are needed in the energy production process. They supply the coenzymes and cofac-tors vital to metabolism of carbohydrates and fats. Vitamins regulate

Table 7.1   Fat Content of Common Protein Foods

Food	Fat calories	Protein calories	Carbohydrate calories
Good choices			
1 cup egg whites	0	102	10
1 cup split peas	18	192	500
1 cup lentils	18	216	456
1 cup red kidney beans	9	168	460
1 cup skim milk	4	34	48
1/4 lb cod (not fried)	9	100	0
1/4 lb tuna (in water)	18	96	0
1/4 lb halibut (not fried)	27	120	0
1/4 lb turkey (no skin)	28	136	0
1/4 lb chicken (no skin)	45	136	0
Moderate choices			
1 cup 1% milk	23	32	45
1 cup 2% milk	45	32	45
1 cup plain yogurt	18	24	30
1/4 lb liver	72	120	24
1/4 lb steak	81	136	0
1 cup cottage cheese	81	100	22
1/4 lb lean ground beef	90	88	0
Not as good choices			
1/4 lb skim milk mozzarella cheese	216	112	14
1 cup hard boiled egg	126	68	6
Poor choices			
1/4 lb pork	225	80	6
4 oz cheddar cheese	252	112	6
1 cup homogenized milk	72	32	44
1 cup scrambled eggs	253	98	19
1/4 lb spare ribs	306	124	0
1/4 lb bologna	324	48	16
1/4 lb salami	360	96	6
1/4 lb bacon	568	138	5

many body functions. Minerals combine to form many body structures and also regulate many body processes. Both are essential for optimal body functioning. However, *excess* vitamins are either stored in fat (fat soluble) or are excreted in the urine (water soluble). A well-balanced, varied diet, selecting foods from all four food groups, will provide all of the vitamins and minerals you need. Excess vitamins and minerals taken as supplements will *not* improve performance, increase energy, increase strength, build more muscle, increase endurance, or prevent sickness. Fruits and vegetables, milk, and meat alternatives (e.g., legumes) are rich in vitamins and minerals. Fats, sugars, and highly processed foods are poor sources of vitamins and minerals.

Vitamin and mineral supplements are not recommended in most situations. Dr. Sue Crawford, sport nutritionist for many international and professional athletes, cautions that "athletes should not allow supplements to give them a false sense of security. They shouldn't think, 'If I eat junk but take my supplements, I'm OK.' Supplements cover only a few of the missing nutrients; you need varied, wholesome food choices to get *all* the nutrients. And supplements can't undo a high-fat, low-fiber, low-water diet."

Water

Water accounts for more than 50 percent of your body weight and is essential to most body functions. It helps regulate body temperature, run the energy production process, and build muscle, and it carries nutrients to body parts while taking waste products away. Sedentary people should drink eight cups of water a day. Athletes who lose a lot of water through sweat during daily practices, games, and workouts need to drink much more water. Refer to pages 183-198 to check exactly when and how much water you should drink.

HEALTHY EATING GUIDELINES

For every advance in sport science and increase in the public's interest in fitness and nutrition, yet another side group emerges to try to profit from myths and misconceptions. Their claims are amazing, stating that without their product, your health or sport performance will surely suffer. They are lying. For long-term health and wellness, along with enhanced sport performance, no product can replace natural food. Here are a few simple guidelines to steer you toward a healthy, balanced diet:

1. Eat a variety of foods to ensure you are getting all of the nutrients your body needs.

2. Select natural foods over processed foods. For example, orange juice is high in carbohydrate, low in fat, and has the vitamin C needed to maintain and repair muscle, cartilage, and bones. OJ also has vitamin A, which strengthens the immune system, and calcium, which has a role in muscle growth and contraction. OJ

contains magnesium, which is involved in blood sugar metabolism, niacin and thiamin, which play a role in the breakdown of carbohydrates, folic acid for growth and development, and phosphorus for nerves and muscles. OJ is a perfect postgame beverage, great for replacing depleted glycogen stores and the water and potassium that have been lost through sweat. Potassium is important to the normal functioning of the heart, muscles, and nervous system. Soft drinks, on the other hand, have no nutrients at all. They are made up of simple sugars and chemicals, and because they have a slight diuretic effect, they are not a good choice for rehydration.

3. Choose food from the vegetables and fruit group and the grain products group more often than foods from the milk products group and meat group.

4. Choose meat alternatives such as legumes, split peas, and kidney beans, which are high in protein and carbohydrate and low in fat.

5. Avoid deep-fried foods and oil-based foods that are high in fat.

6. When preparing meals, cook from scratch. Steam, barbecue, broil, bake, or microwave foods rather than frying. Steaming food retains nutrients better than any other cooking method.

7. Many foods are fine to eat raw, which of course leaves all nutrients intact and adds no fat. Green peppers, red potatoes, and carrots, for example, taste good when raw and are highly portable foods—quick and easy for packing in a lunch when you're on the go. Eat them just like you would an apple or banana. Don't let societal norms dictate which foods are okay to pack up and eat uncooked—let your taste buds and health interests decide. Skip the drive-through lane, and make raw fruits and vegetables your choice for "fast food." A raw red potato is 90 percent carbohydrate—an excellent energy food. French fries are over 50 percent fat.

8. Don't let society tell you what types of foods are OK to eat at certain meal times. You want to eat healthy foods that you enjoy and that provide energy for hockey. Go ahead and eat a thick-crust vegetarian pizza for breakfast. Try oatmeal for lunch. Cereal with skim milk and a sliced banana, toast and jam, and orange juice is great for postpractice refueling. You shouldn't follow what past generations commonly ate at each meal. Eat what is right for you today.

9. Consistently plan your food intake ahead of time—but don't restrict yourself to a category. You don't have to be a vegetarian. Just try overall to eat low-fat, healthy foods the majority of the time. Plan your groceries, home meals, packed lunches, and

restaurant meals so that you are eating the right foods at the right times to fuel and refuel your body pre- and postactivity. Don't find yourself out at meal times (or snack times) without having planned what you're going to eat. Preferably have it with you. Spontaneous meals are often high in fat and low in nutrients, such as chocolate bars or cheeseburgers and fries.

10. There are many *minor* food alterations that will lower the fat content without having to eliminate the entire food. For instance, trading one ingredient or topping for another (e.g., on sub sandwiches, substituting turkey for pepperoni, mustard for mayonnaise, and skim milk cheese for regular cheese) can make a significant difference in the fat content while allowing you to still enjoy the same foods. When you select low-fat main food items, don't ruin the good choice by adding high-fat, low-nutrient toppings and spreads.

When cooking at home, try experimenting with common recipes. You'll discover that you can eliminate most oils and cut down on butter and margarine, and often your food will end up tasting just as good or better. Many high-fat ingredients in recipes are either not really needed or not needed in the volume the recipe calls for.

Enjoy eating well. Like exercise, it makes you feel better. Just as you've learned to appreciate your body's response to a workout, notice the effects of healthy eating on your overall mood and attitude. Get into the positive cycle of eating to feel good.

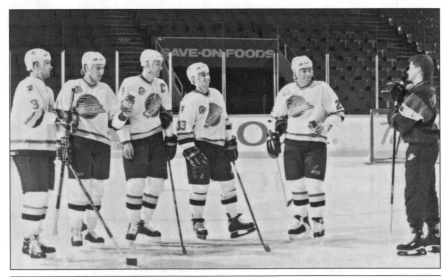

Bret Hedican, Jyrki Lumme, Trevor Linden, Mike Peca, Jeff Brown, and Pete Twist stop for fluid replenishment before the next drill.

CARBOHYDRATE: THE MASTER SPORT FUEL

Carbohydrate is the preferred fuel for intense hockey action. Skating, shooting, and bodychecking all consume carbohydrates. Most carbohydrates in your body are stored in muscles as muscle glycogen, and a bit in the liver, which is used to maintain a healthy blood sugar level. Muscle glycogen supplies the energy for playing hockey, but it is only stored in limited amounts. Even the leanest NHL player has over 30 times the calories stored as fat than he does carbohydrates. Since carbohydrate stores are relatively small, and hockey preferentially uses carbohydrates for energy, players need repetitive refueling, eating carbohydrates each day and each meal.

Preventing fatigue is critical to allowing hockey skills and technique to proceed unimpeded. When your muscles run out of glycogen, your legs feel tired. Players may experience this in the third period, if they have not eaten properly on the days preceding the game. Once fatigued, players lose speed, strength, and stride power; their skating ability and technique is adversely affected. After the muscles' supply of glycogen is depleted, the body turns to the liver for glycogen. This results in low blood sugar, which causes mental fatigue and lethargy—not quite the best condition for a hockey game!

Since the intensity of most games increases as the game progresses, a player's ability to give 100 percent late in the third period is critical to the team's success or failure. The ability for intense physical performance becomes severely limited when energy stores are depleted. Consequently, your goal is to plan ahead and have as much muscle glycogen as possible during the third period of a game or in the latter stages of intense off-ice conditioning. There are two ways to increase your storage of glycogen: conditioning and carbohydrate loading.

Conditioning

Adaptations to on-ice and off-ice conditioning include increasing the amount of glycogen that your body makes naturally and stores in your muscles. Nutrition and training go hand in hand. Proper nutrition allows hockey players to train harder and longer. And well-conditioned athletes can then store more carbohydrates. Once they can store more carbohydrates, they can train with an even greater volume. And the cycle continues. During early season exhibitions, some players simply cannot compete at a high intensity throughout the game. By the end of the season, most players can play full-out in the third period and even into overtime. This is partly because their bodies have become able to store greater amounts of glycogen. So, workouts are not just to develop the fitness, strength, speed, and energy systems needed for hockey performance. While physical development will in itself give you more stamina, the workout is also telling your body to store more glycogen, which will also increase your endurance. You'll have a double advantage over less prepared players.

Carbohydrate Loading

Carbohydrate loading was originally a nutritional strategy used successfully in sports that have fewer competition days and more training or practice days. For a track and field athlete keying in on a one-day competition, a true carbohydrate loading system may require several days. First, the athlete's activity level is increased for three days and carbohydrate intake is reduced, depleting glycogen stores. Then activity is tapered down over three days while carbohydrate intake is maximized, resulting in a supercompensation affect (greater glycogen storage than normally achieved).

Hockey players need to carbohydrate load every single day. Elite players have daily practices and games, plus off-ice practices to develop strength, power, endurance, speed, agility, and flexibility. Younger players face a similar, though less intense, schedule but also have other sportsthey are involved in. To meet the energy requirements and recover from the high volume of activity, players need to consume a diet high in carbohydrates every day, both before and after games and practices. See table 7.2 for a list of foods high in carbohydrates and low in fat.

Throughout a season, coaches typically target game days when scheduling high-carbohydrate meals. But while some players see 20 to 30 minutes of ice time per game, many others range from 0 to 10 minutes. But on practice days *all* players skate for 60 to 90 minutes, plus complete off-ice conditioning and participate in other activities. In this way, game days may be overemphasized as a nutritional concern. It is equally or even more important to consume carbohydrates on practice days. The bottom line is that hockey players—from young aspiring athletes to veteran professional players—need to "carbo load" each and every day.

There are several guidelines for loading the body with energy before a hockey game. If a game is on Friday, emphasize eating high-carbohydrate meals on Wednesday and Thursday, so that the glycogen stores are already being filled. Glycogen storage, in the face of daily activity, is a continual process that cannot be completed in one sitting on

Table 7.2 High-Carbohydrate and Low-Fat Food Sources

Food source	Carbohydrate calories	Fat calories
Good choices		
Fruits		
1 cup dates	520	9
1 cup raisins	448	0
1 cup sweetened applesauce	244	0
1 cup pineapple	240	0
1 cup apple/orange juice	120	0
1 banana	108	0
1 orange	100	0
1 cup blueberries	88	0
1 apple	84	0
1/2 cantaloupe	80	0
1 cup grapes	64	0
1 cup strawberries	48	0
Vegetables		
1 cup corn	168	0
1 baked potato	128	0
1 cup peas	76	0
Grain products		
1 bagel	180	9
1 cup rice	180	0
Bran muffin	180	36
1 cup raisin bran	168	9
1 cup dried fruit mix	160	0
Frosted pop tarts	152	45
1 cup egg noodles	148	18
2 slices pumpernickel bread	136	9
1 cup spaghetti with tomato sauce	136	9
Instant oatmeal cereal	120	18
2 slices rye bread	104	9
2 slices whole wheat bread	96	18
2 pancakes	96	27
1 tbsp honey	68	0
1 tbsp jam	20	0
Meat alternatives		
1 cup dried split peas	500	18
1 cup red kidney beans	460	9
1 cup lentils	456	18

(continued)

Table 7.2 *(continued)*

Food source	Carbohydrate calories	Fat calories
Not as good choices		
1/4 lb bacon	5	568
1/4 lb sausage	16	494
1/4 lb salami	6	360
1/4 lb bologna	16	324
1/4 lb spareribs	0	306
1/4 lb pork	6	225
1/4 lb steak	0	81
4 oz potato chips	220	405
4 oz onion rings	160	270
4 oz mozzarella cheese	14	216
4 oz hash browns	48	144
4 oz french fries	90	100
1 cup whole milk	44	72

Friday. Come game day, players should have a high-carbohydrate breakfast, taking some of the pressure off of getting all their energy from the pregame meal. For the pregame meal, there are several specific food selection and timing guidelines that will help maximize glycogen levels and optimize on-ice performance.

PREGAME NUTRITION

You used to hear stories of players sitting down for pregame meals of big steaks, deep-fried foods, and potatoes smothered in butter, sour cream, and bacon bits. Maybe a heavy shake to wash it all down. Such stories amaze me, but I know they're true because I ate such meals. As a young minor league hockey player, I was given by my coaches a couple of chocolate bars 20 minutes before a game for "instant energy." The steaks and high-fat foods didn't digest well or provide any energy. The chocolate bars made me dizzy and lethargic.

Today, the science of nutrition can provide athletes with amazing tools to assist their game performance. After 14 years in the NHL and a Stanley Cup Championship with the New York Rangers, Steve Larmer recognizes the power of nutrition:

> Players' food intake has changed from my rookie season to today. Cutting a lot of fat out of the diet, and just staying away from junk food like potato chips, chocolate, and other foods

that aren't really healthy for you. Once in a while it's fine to have a little treat, but not as part of your daily intake. We eat a lot of foods that are high in carbohydrate, like pasta and potatoes. Everyone is cutting back on their red meat. It all helps, both with maintaining your playing weight and trying to get as much energy as you can out of the food you eat. If you're not eating a balanced diet that consists of high-carbohydrate sources including a lot of vegetables and fruits, your body's not going to be able to perform at the level it's capable of.

The Pregame Meal

Five to six hours before a game, eat a large meal high in carbohydrates and low in fat and protein. Carbohydrates top off your hockey fuel tanks and are more easily digested than fat and protein foods. Five hours leaves enough time for digestion but is not so long that you'll be overly hungry when you step onto the ice. If the food has not digested, it will not be available for energy. Additionally, only 20 percent of the normal blood will be available at the stomach to continue digestion because the body is diverting oxygen to your skating muscles. This slows the digestion process. There is a misconception that you want the stomach empty to allow oxygenated blood to go to the working muscles. The oxygenated blood will go to the muscles anyway to meet the demands of skating and bodychecking. This is why you get stomach cramps with food left in the stomach slowly digesting. Select pregame foods you are familiar with so that you know your taste buds will allow you to eat an adequate amount, and you know the food's effect on your body—this is not the time to try the spicy bean dip for the first time.

A pregame snack three hours before the game will supply a little more energy and prevent hunger pains during the game. The closer you get to game time, the lighter (i.e., less fat, protein, and fiber) and more liquid the food. A pregame snack should be foods like yogurt, fruit juice, bananas, bagels, and low-fiber cereal and skim milk. Whether you eat this snack or not really depends on personal preference. Some of my players eat a big pregame meal, rest or sleep, get up and go to the rink. Others have the big pregame meal plus a small snack later in the afternoon (for a 7:30 night game). When players experiment with exact timing, food choices, and amount consumed, they should do this during the off-season or on practice days—not on game days.

Game Day Bus Trips

I'm 12. I wake up at 6:00 A.M. to eat a quick breakfast Mom got up early to prepare. Dad drops me off at the rink, and I board the team bus. Five hours later, we arrive at our destination, the opposition's town, 90 minutes before game time. Driving through town on the way to the rink, we stop at McDonalds and bring some food back onto the bus. We gobble down our meals—high protein, super-high fat—food that will supply very little energy and take a long time to digest. We arrive at the arena as I try to quickly finish my cheeseburger and fries. Picking up my three sticks and equipment bag from the bus storage, I enter the rink carrying sticks and bag in one hand so I can hold my milkshake in the other hand. The results of this are horrendous, but playing on an empty stomach is not an option, so what is a practical solution?

To avoid buses littered with pop cans, chip bags, and candy bar wrappers, and to eliminate the fast food stop, coaches must emphasize to parents the importance of having high-carbohydrate meals the day before the game and during breakfast the day of the game. Get the parents involved, packing high-carbohydrate, low-fat sandwiches with thick slices of whole wheat bread. Include lots of bottled water (still a lot cheaper than fast food), canned juices, fresh fruit, raisins and other dried fruit, and bagels with honey and jams. Satisfy the players' taste buds while supplying the carbohydrates and fluids they need. Keep the food in coolers, and pass out food at a designated time for a *team* meal right on the bus. This saves time, money, and provides the nutrients needed for hockey. When it becomes a formal part of the team's schedule, and players realize the timing of this meal and the food made available is designed to help them improve their on-ice performance, it will soon become a standard part of their game preparation. Eating a "game preparation" meal together on the bus will also get them thinking about the game earlier.

This setup may also help expose more parents to sport nutrition guidelines, which may result in their providing better pregame meals for home games, too. Parents play a very major role in hockey nutrition. If there's not an assistant coach who can structure the team's game preparation nutrition, place a couple of parents in charge of organizing bus meals and educational handouts for all parents. Most teams will have a player's parent who is well read on nutrition, or who adopts a healthy diet for fitness or lifestyle reasons. Whether through team meetings or by getting the players involved in designing team meals and educational handouts, make sure players understand how specific food selections will help their athletic performance.

It is important to eat vegetables each day, including game day. Vegetables supply the vitamins and minerals vital to the energy production process. Without them, the body is unable to use all of the glycogen stored in the muscles. Think of pumping a car full of high premium gasoline but then not adding oil to the engine—your car won't run, and all that good fuel goes to waste!

Last Minute Energy?

Eating or drinking a carbohydrate source (e.g., fruit juice) or simple sugar (e.g., candy) for "quick energy" within 60 minutes of the game can have a negative effect. Such consumption rapidly boosts your blood glucose, giving you an initial energy burst, but it also triggers insulin to transport excess glucose out of the blood and into the muscles and fat cells. Combined with exercise, your blood glucose level can drop, leaving you feeling lethargic, fatigued, weak, or lightheaded. This rapid drop in blood glucose is called *hypoglycemia*. Eating carbohydrates within an hour of exercise causes blood insulin levels to triple, causing blood glucose to be less available, which places greater dependence on muscle glycogen stores to supply the energy for hockey. Consequently, muscle glycogen stores are depleted faster, and you fatigue sooner. Insulin also blocks the utilization of fat, so even easy, submaximal efforts have to be fueled by carbohydrates. This further speeds glycogen use.

More research is needed on this topic. Some sport scientists are proposing that carbohydrate consumption soon before a game may not be the problem we thought it was. Some recent studies support the traditional thinking that such consumption can cause serious problems, but other studies show no positive or negative effects. Still others report positive energy-enhancing effects. Dr. Ted Rhodes at the University of British Columbia is examining ingestion of carbohydrates 10 minutes prior to exercise. At this point, it's enough that you're forewarned of the

Table 7.3   Pregame Meal Guidelines

High carbohydrate
Low fat
Low protein
Plenty of water and juice
5 to 6 hours before game
Stick with familiar foods
Eat easily digestible foods

possible side-effects. Likely, there are individual differences in how bodies respond to "quick energy." Until more information is available, I recommend avoiding carbohydrate sources within 60 minutes of a game. If you must experiment, do it on practice days.

Pregame Fluids

Water is an important nutrient for both health and sport performance. One of water's roles is to regulate body temperature. Excess heat is dissipated in the form of sweat, and the body cools when the sweat evaporates. During a hockey game, your need for energy increases, so your fuel is burned at a faster rate. When fuel is burned to release energy for the muscle contractions that allow you to skate, a great deal of excess heat is given off. The rate of heat production by active muscles can be 100 times that of inactive muscles, so cooling is again very important. For the body's cooling system to work effectively, you need to maintain an adequate fluid level.

Water is also required for the chemical reactions in the muscles that release energy for movement. This is why muscle tissue has a higher water content than fat tissue—because more water is required to carry out the chemical reactions involved in the vigorous function of the muscle. Water is also a key ingredient of blood volume, so the heart, lungs, and entire circulatory system depend on your body's water level.

Table 7.4   Ten-Step Nutrition Plan for a Friday 7:30 P.M. Game

---

1. Day to day and week to week, eat a well-balanced, healthy, low-fat, varied diet.
2. Carbo load Wednesday and Thursday, plus eat a variety of vegetables.
3. Carbohydrate breakfast Friday morning, plus plenty of fluids.
4. Pregame meal, 1:30 P.M. Friday.
    High-carbohydrate, low-fat, low-protein foods
    Plenty of fluids (water and juice)
5. Optional: Pregame carbohydrate snack at about 4:30 P.M.
6. Drink water up until 6:00 P.M.
7. *No* complex carbohydrates or simple sugars in last hour before game time.
8. During game: Continually sip water or carbohydrate in solution, as much as you can tolerate.
9. Postgame: Consume a moderate amount of fruit, juice, and bagels *immediately* after the game
10. Eat a full carbohydrate meal 1 to $1^1/_2$ hours after the game.

The rate of sweating during a game will vary from player to player and also depend on work intensity and temperature and humidity in the arena. Prepare ahead for the fluids that will be lost through sweat by consuming plenty of water on the days before a game. Your kidneys need 60 to 90 minutes to process excess liquid, so stop drinking fluids 90 minutes before game time to allow the excess to be eliminated through the urine before game time. Drink one to two cups of water 5 to 10 minutes before your game to add a little extra fluid to help replace sweat losses.

NUTRITION DURING THE GAME

As muscle glycogen stores are depleted, your body gets more energy from blood glucose, which is transported from the blood into the skating, shooting, and bodychecking muscles. Ingesting liquid carbohydrates throughout the game will help ensure enough carbohydrate is available for energy late in the third period. Don't wait for the third period to think about replacing carbohydrates—begin in the first period. Once the game has started, drinking small amounts of carbohydrate does not cause hypoglycemia. (Exercise suppresses insulin release and prevents rebound hypoglycemia.) The carbohydrate taken during the game can be used as energy. Commercial sport drinks are helpful during a game, when you want a diluted source of carbohydrate. Sport drinks offer the percentage of carbohydrate in solution (6 to 8 percent) that allows for fast emptying from the stomach, so the fluid and carbohydrate is readily available to replace sweat losses and boost blood glucose levels. More concentrated drinks are slow to leave the stomach and are a poor game choice.

Fluid Intake

If you do not replace the fluids you lose as sweat, you dehydrate and your blood volume decreases. This affects blood circulation, and blood supply to the muscles shuts down, destroying your ability to maintain athletic effort. The muscles you are asking to perform for you on the ice cannot receive the volume of oxygen they need to function because your body preferentially keeps the limited blood volume for the heart and lungs.

It seems simple enough that you should drink some water or juice when you feel thirsty. Thirst is triggered by a high concentration of sodium in the blood. When you sweat, you lose water from the blood (part of the cooling process). Then the remaining blood is more concentrated with sodium (because of the lowered water content). This triggers the thirst mechanism and increases your desire to drink. But by the time the brain discovers this and sends the message that you are thirsty, you've already lost 1 percent of your body weight. For a 200-pound player, this is 2 pounds, or four cups of water. If this player does not take in fluids, water loss can quickly progress to 2 percent (4 pounds, or eight cups of water) and at this point work capacity is diminished by 15 percent, severely hampering hockey performance.

Thirst is *not* a good indicator of your water needs. God didn't create the thirst mechanism for optimal hockey performance. It is there for survival—to protect us in extreme situations. To prevent dehydration during games, drink well *before* you are thirsty. Your body takes in and retains water at a slower rate than it loses fluids through sweat. So, to prevent falling too far behind your body's water needs, and to prevent dehydration, begin drinking water right at the beginning of the first period.

I've had players drink water before and during a game and still drop 5 percent of their body weight to fluids lost through sweat, so I cannot emphasize enough the importance of water intake. Try to drink water throughout the game, between shifts and periods. Drink as much as you can without causing stomach discomfort.

POSTGAME NUTRITION

I've had goaltenders who play a full 60 minutes and lose up to 10 pounds by the end of a game. This weight drop is water loss, not fat loss. A lot of water is lost to sweat over the course of a hockey game. The intense physical activity, extra weight of protective equipment, arena lights, and humidity from the fans all contribute to hockey players sweating profusely.

As a general rule, for every pound of weight loss after a game, you need to drink two cups of fluid. Pregame and postgame weigh-ins indicate how much replacement fluid is needed. Your urine also provides feedback. Clear urine indicates normal water balance. Dark urine indicates a concentration of metabolic wastes and that more water is needed. Some vitamin supplements also turn the urine yellow (but not as dark), so if you're taking vitamin supplements, urine color is a less reliable indicator. In this case, you can assess your body water level by

Postgame Meals

Many coaches have presented the postgame meal as a problem for young teams that face both a long bus ride home immediately after the game and also budget restrictions. Coaches can have home-prepared food and drinks packed on the bus to save time and money while ensuring a healthy, high-carbohydrate post-game meal. Coaches can also stop the bus at a grocery store to allow players to pick up some food and drink items. A convenience store presents mainly junk food options. A grocery store has a great variety of easily portable, highly-carbohydrate foods—fruit, breads, pretzels, pop tarts, drinks, raisins, and the like.

McDonalds type fast food restaurants seem to be a regular post-game stop for a quick meal before a long bus ride. This is a worst case scenario nutritionally. If occasionally it is the only option, I recommend coaches at least provide juice and fruit and bagels in the dressing room and use the 20-minute window of opportunity immediately after the game. This way, the players' sport nutrition is partially taken care of be-fore they eat their high-fat, nutritionally empty fast food. They first received some healthy carbohydrates and got a good start to glycogen replenishment. Moreover, they won't be as hungry when it comes time to select meals at the fast food restaurant.

If a restaurant meal is required, coaches can set up a much better situation. Coaches should determine where the team will eat *before* leaving for the roadtrip. During the first visit to each opponent's town, coaches can take the time to look for a suitable restaurant. It's important to develop a working relationship with the restaurant manager. The restaurant will appreciate the team's regular business and will usually be amenable to serving special foods that are requested ahead of time. The menu available to the players is preestablished with the restaurant, and an approximate arrival time is confirmed. After the game, players' options for food intake is well structured for optimal hockey nutrition, and the food is ready quickly. For even more time efficiency, the players can preselect their meals before the game, so it's ready when they arrive at the restaurant. A mini-buffet at the restaurant is another good solution. This allows a greater volume of carbohydrate intake, and the meal is ready as soon as the team arrives at the restaurant.

With all of the above options, a team should be able to negotiate a very reasonable price (definitely no more than a fast food bill), especially if there are over 20 people and it becomes the team's regular stop. This way, the coach will know the type and timing of postgame food before the team even leaves for the roadtrip.

the quantity and smell of your urine. If volume is less than normal for you and you detect an ammonia smell, you need to drink more water. The best sources of water are plain water (filtered, bottled, or spring) and juices. Caffeinated pop, iced-tea, and alcoholic drinks slow rehydration and recovery.

Postgame carbohydrates are even more important than your pregame meal. Immediately after intense activity, you have 20 minutes when your muscles are most receptive to taking in carbohydrates and storing them as muscle glycogen. Think of it as the door to your muscles being wide open for 20 minutes. As a general rule, the sooner the better. A banana and two cans of juice during these 20 minutes replenish a lot of muscle fuel. If you don't take advantage of this 20-minute window, it will take you longer to get your energy stores up to the same level. If you have a game the next night, or a hard practice the next day, you won't have enough time to get your stores up as high as the athlete who takes advantage of the 20-minute window—no matter how much pasta and other carbohydrates you eat afterward!

That the optimal time for replenishing occurs immediately after a game or practice works out perfectly for coaches of young teams. Once players leave the arena, coaches have no control over what they eat. But to take advantage of the 20-minute window, carbohydrates must be consumed right in the dressing room. Have specific foods and drinks laid out in the dressing room area. Following a game, the first thing my players do when they get off the ice is reach for a juice drink or carbohydrate drink, a piece of fruit, or a bagel.

Sport drinks that are water with 6 to 8 percent carbohydrate in solution can help the fluid and carbohydrate replenishment process. But don't depend on only sport drinks for postgame recovery. Fruit and juice are better choices. They offer more healthy nutrients in addition to carbohydrates and water. Plus, after the game, you should select full-strength, carbohydrate-rich beverages and foods to replace the glycogen burned during the game. In comparison, sport drinks are more suited for *during* the game, not after. Plain water is also necessary to help restore the body's fluid balance.

Optimize absorption of liquid carbohydrate sources by following the five simple guidelines in table 7.5.

The Postgame Meal

After players have left the rink, they should eat a full postgame meal one to two hours later. This meal is similar to the pregame meal, consisting

Table 7.5   Fluid Replenishment Guidelines

1. Volume	Drink as much as tolerable.
2. Temperature	Cold is better. Cold fluid absorbs into the small intestine better. You will drink a greater volume of fluid when it is cold and you'll drink it more quickly.
3. Concentration of glucose in water	6 to 12% CHO in solution absorbs well, while 20% (e.g., oranges) is too high and decreases absorption rate. Lower concentrations are used during the game while higher concentrations are better postgame.
4. Sodium	Assists with water absorption.
5. Taste	Provide athletes with flavors they like so they will drink more.

of carbohydrates, fruits and vegetables, and fluids. Refueling not only depends on the amount of carbohydrates and the timing of carbohydrate consumption but is also affected by the food's *glycemic index*. Carbohydrates can be categorized as having low, moderate, or high glycemic levels. High-glycemic foods are converted to blood glucose and transported to the muscles at a faster rate than low-glycemic foods. This is significant after exercise and after games, when athletes are trying to speed up the recovery of muscle glycogen. Hockey players can become glycogen-depleted after one intense game, or from progressive depletion following a heavy game schedule and repetitive practices. Eating high-glycemic carbohydrates at key times will help speed up and maximize refueling. Table 7.6 lists some moderate- and high-glycemic foods that increase the rate of glycogen replenishment.

PRACTICE INTENSITY, GAME SCHEDULE, AND ENERGY DEPLETION

A last word on progressive glycogen depletion: Say a team has games on Wednesday and Friday night. If they play poorly on Wednesday, a common coach reaction is to punish the team with extra physical work at practice on Thursday, skating players until they drop. The coach declares that the team has to get "in shape" for Friday's game. But athletes cannot get in shape in one day. What they'll do on Thursday is further deplete their energy stores, making it far less likely that they'll play well Friday. Even if players are physically, mentally, and emotionally willing to give their all, they will not perform well because they

Table 7.6   Glycemic Index for Postgame Carbohydrates

High-glycemic foods	Moderate-glycemic foods	Low-glycemic foods
Honey	Corn	Apples
Sugar	Grapes	Dates
Bagels	Oranges	Milk
Bread	Spaghetti	Yogurt
Raisins	Rye bread	Beans
Potatoes	Oatmeal	Lentils
	Rice	

won't have enough fuel for three intense periods of hockey. So, following Wednesday's poor performance, the coach is better off scheduling a *light* practice on Thursday. You can spend the rest of the time giving the players concrete feedback, which they always appreciate. Show them where they went wrong in the bad game, teach technique, systems, and positioning—things players can *think* about that will help their play on Friday. A light practice does not have to be an ineffective practice. You can work on quickness and agility drills that are intense but very short in duration—these will not use up a lot of energy and are fun to do, creating an atmosphere in which players enjoy hockey. At the same time, emphasize carbohydrate loading. With the combination of a tough game Wednesday, a light practice Thursday, and carbohydrate loading Thursday (and Friday pregame), players approach Friday's game mentally more prepared, having *learned* on Thursday, and their energy stores will be topped up or even supercompensated at 20 percent above normal, as opposed to entering Friday's game tired and depleted.

WEIGHT GAIN

There are hockey players at all levels who are interested in gaining lean muscle mass. They are striving to improve size, strength, dynamic balance, stride power, bodychecking, injury prevention, speed, quickness, agility, and shooting. All of these physical skills and technical skills can be improved by first building a solid base of lean muscle mass. Joe Murphy of the Chicago Black Hawks increased his weight by 15 pounds in 1994, which helped his goal production. He explains, "Before, if a player would get a hand or stick on me, I'd had it. Now I can go right through them."

All-Day Tournaments and Back-to-Back Games

Minor hockey teams enter tournaments in which they may play two or three games in one day. Teams at *all* levels face back-to-back games (games on successive nights). The goal is to try to delay fatigue so players still have some energy during the last period of the last game. Working hard all day or on repetitive days results in a progressive depletion of muscle glycogen. It takes 24 to 48 hours to top off muscle glycogen stores. This is why coaches may structure an intense practice one day but an easy practice the next day. Even if eating properly, without light days or rest days, the player's energy stores are progressively lowered each day.

To prepare for all-day tournaments or back-to-back games, the last two practice days should be fairly light, while players carbo load every meal. The day of the first game, players should get up early enough to eat a high-carbohydrate breakfast. Extra sleep won't do much good if the player runs out of fuel.

Liquid carbohydrate sources on the bench will allow players to sip a bit between each shift. This will be used for energy during the game, helping to preserve muscle glycogen stores.

After each game, there should be carbohydrate sources available in the dressing room—juice, fruit, bagels, sport drinks—so all players can take advantage of the "20-minute window of opportunity." At all-day tournaments, there is obviously not enough time to eat and fully digest a restaurant meal before the next game. The dressing room carbohydrates provide immediate carbohydrate replenishment, plus are of a small enough volume so that digestion should be complete before the next game. Coaches should also have plenty of cold water available in the dressing room to aid fluid replenishment. After leaving the dressing room, if players want a snack, they should have prepacked snacks from home. Athletic competitions, oddly enough, usually offer food such as pop, french fries, hamburgers, hot dogs, and potato chips, all high-fat, low-nutrient sources that take a long time to digest. So, come prepared with dressing room food and snacks from home to maximize those hockey fuel tanks!

An average draft pick reporting for his first NHL training camp weighs less than the veteran players but has a higher percentage of body fat. This means the draft pick has much less muscle mass and more fat. Likely, this young player has tried to increase his weight to improve performance and help him handle the bigger NHL players. "Early in my career, the biggest thing that changed my game was my fitness level," declares Geoff Courtnall of the St. Louis Blues. "One summer, I just totally dedicated myself to five days of training each week—weights, running, riding, and just making a commitment. Not only did I get in great shape, but I gained 20 pounds. I think that was probably the turning point in my career, where I had that extra step and seemed to be that much ahead of players in training camp. That was the best camp I had, as well as the best year."

Diet Guidelines for Gaining Lean Muscle

At any age group, whenever a player moves up a level, the average player will be bigger. To increase lean muscle mass without adding fat, nutrition and strength training must be completed together. For more information on strength training, see the sidebar on page 201 and chapter 4. Weight gain—specifically, gain of lean muscle tissue—can be accomplished by following the diet and exercise guidelines below.

1. Increase your daily caloric intake to consume more calories than you're expending. You'll need additional food to meet the caloric demands of heavy muscle-building workouts, plus more food on top of that. On average, to gain a pound a week, you need to consume 500 additional calories a day. This is 500 calories over and above the added calories you need for the extra strength training workouts.
2. Eat as large a portion as you can tolerate each meal.
3. Eat five meals a day (three big meals and two snacks). Adopt a "grazing" approach.
4. Eat a big breakfast every day.
5. Eat or drink a late night snack. Blended drinks work well after your last meal or before going to bed.
6. Look at food as your *weight gain medicine*. Do not skip a meal, even if you're not hungry! Remind yourself you have to take your medicine!
7. Select foods high in calories. Some players get sick of eating so much. It becomes a real chore. If they can pick a food that is more

dense with calories, they'll be taking in calories more efficiently and won't have to eat so much. Two foods of the same type (e.g., fruit) may be the same size and take the same amount of time to eat, but one may have twice the calories. Keep eating healthy, low-fat foods, but select *denser* foods. For example, pineapples, raisins, and bananas contain more calories than watery fruits like grape-fruit and peaches. When choosing a soup, go for barley, lentil, or split pea—they have more calories than chicken or tomato. For sandwiches, select hearty breads such as rye or pumpernickel, as opposed to light fluffy breads.

8. Be patient and consistent.

9. Add high-calorie (but low-fat) toppings and spreads and ingredients to your foods. You can add a great number of calories by adding onto foods you are eating. Skim milk powder, jams, honey, breadcrumbs, chopped walnuts, parmesan cheese, and cottage cheese are just a few extra toppings that you can add to foods without excessively increasing your fat intake.

10. Increase your carbohydrate intake, without increasing your protein or fat intake. Additional carbohydrates are required to fuel the heavy workouts needed to build muscle mass and put on weight.

If it takes longer than you think it should to gain weight, be patient and continue the steps listed above. Don't spend money on protein supplements or weight gain formulas. Protein is required for growth and repair of muscle tissue, but most people get more protein than they need from their regular food intake and even more when on a high caloric weight gain diet. Excess protein is not stored as muscle. Extra protein is either sent to the kidneys and excreted through the urine, or is stored as fat. Strength and lean mass building workouts require a lot of energy—if you're eating too much protein, you're doing so at the expense of carbohydrates. You're being filled up by protein and eating less carbohydrate foods, so you won't maximize your energy stores. And you won't be supplying your body with the energy needed for high-volume, high-intensity, lean mass building workouts—so your muscles do not develop as much. *Exercise* builds bigger muscles, not excess protein. Carbohydrates also indirectly promote muscle growth. When carbohydrates enter the blood stream, insulin is released to increase muscle permeability to glycogen, so the muscles will take up and store glycogen. The released insulin also increases amino acid uptake by the muscles. Carbohydrates cause the insulin release, which promotes the synthesis of muscle protein and reduces muscle protein breakdown.

Diet Supplements and Weight Gain Formulas: Don't Be Duped!

Protein supplements, amino acid supplements, and most other "miracle" methods of gaining weight are a waste of money. As I just mentioned, extra protein will not help you gain the lean mass you want. Additionally, the protein in natural food protein sources is assimilated much better than protein supplements. Your body does not even take in and use much of the protein from supplements. As for amino acids, they are simply the "building blocks" of protein. If you're eating a well-balanced diet, you'll be getting all the amino acids you need. There is no supplement that provides a magical amino acid that food does not provide.

Supplement companies typically extract one line from a research paper that, out of context, sounds like it supports their product. They highlight that line in their advertising. Or they conduct their own research, and highlight *one* subject who gained lean mass when taking their supplement. I can take an athlete and have him easily gain 10 pounds of lean muscle mass just with specific exercise and natural food—so it is no surprise that a subject who is taking a company's supplement while strength training and eating proper food will gain weight!

Supplement companies refer to "growth hormone," which stimulates muscle growth. A common advertisement is the effect of amino acids on growth hormone. *Arginine* is one amino acid common in supplements that supposedly stimulates the release of growth hormone. But amino acids taken orally do not result in an elevated growth hormone concentration greater than the level caused by exercise alone! To elevate growth hormone levels more than exercise does, you would need to consume at least 30 amino acid tablets at once. (Don't do this!)

Examine weight gain formulas. Many of them list skim milk powder as their main ingredient. You're better off saving your money and buying a big bag of skim milk powder from a grocery store and using it as a base for homemade blender drinks. The funny thing about some manufacturers' weight gain and weight loss powders is that they have the *same* ingredients. The only difference is the instructions. For the weight gain powder, they tell you to take it in addition to your regular meals. For the weight loss powder, they tell you to take it in place of meals!

Protein supplements may be advertised as "hydrolyzed," which they say means predigested, so your body won't have to spend any energy on digestion. But why pay 20 to 30 times the cost of natural foods for predigested protein supplements when your body was specifically designed to break down and digest food! Such supplements are just a new angle to create a supposed need for a product.

Exercise Guidelines For Gaining Lean Muscle

1. Use strength training as your main exercise. Intense strength training produces the best muscle growth results.
2. Use heavy weights and low (six) reps per set. Through trial and error, select a weight that causes fatigue after the sixth rep.
3. Use a high volume (large number of sets) workout.
4. Select exercise with multijoint movements.
5. Use strict technique for safety and optimal results. Sacrificing technique in order to lift heavier weights will result in less muscle growth.
6. Progressively increase the weight to keep working the muscle hard as you get stronger. You must maximally overload the muscle to stimulate growth.
7. Use slow eccentric contractions, called "negatives," with a 1:4 positive-negative ratio of movement. This means taking one second for the positive phase of the lift, and four seconds for the negative phase of the lift. The muscle is working harder during the negative phase, promoting greater muscle adaptations.
8. Complete forced reps: Use a spotter to help you force out one or two extra reps after you are too fatigued to complete any more reps on your own. During the last couple of reps, the muscle must recruit more and more motor units to handle the same weight. The muscle effectively works harder on the last reps, stimulating more growth.
9. Allow at least 36 hours rest between strength training sessions for each muscle group.
10. Be patient. Weight gain is a process that continues through to mid- to late twenties for many players. Along the way, emphasize performance gains. Even if you only gain a couple of pounds, at the very least you'll have improved your strength and sport performance.

Many athletes do find it difficult to gain weight. Indeed, even some fully mature athletes have a hard time just maintaining their weight in the face of daily conditioning, practices, and games. For these players, some commercial powders might be useful. For example, our team uses Musashi products with some players to complement their exercise and nutrition weight gain programs. These contain complex carbohydrate sources to help boost energy stores, along with some high quality protein. Being able to add on to their meals an easily consumed liquid, high-calorie drink seems perfect for these players. They are most often utilized postpractice, when players can more easily tolerate cold liquid carbohydrate sources. At home, players can also mix ice cubes, skim milk, skim milk powder, egg whites, bananas, and low-fat ice cream with frozen strawberries or raspberries for a delicious and refreshing, high-carbohydrate, high-protein, high-calorie, high-nutrient, low-fat, cost-effective drink.

CHAPTER 8

CONDITIONING FOR EVERY SEASON

You have a lot to accomplish: aerobic conditioning, building the anaerobic energy systems, developing strength, power, and muscular endurance, conditioning quickness and agility, developing speed, and improving flexibility. All of these must complement one another, plus support hockey skill development and specifically improve game performance. Player development can't be accomplished piecemeal. All physical components have to be conditioned in light of one another—certain ones need to be developed before others can build off of them; some need to be worked while others rest.

When designing a year-round conditioning program, it's important first to know your current status of hockey fitness. Fitness testing will not only help identify players' strengths and weaknesses, it will also allow you to judge the effectiveness of your training program.

ASSESSING HOCKEY CONDITIONING

Physiological assessments can be used to rank and compare players, or to identify what fitness components each player needs to work on. Test results offer players an objective evaluation of their conditioning and help motivate them to improve their performance levels. A test-retest approach helps the coach track each individual's progress. Ideally, the testing protocol should be as specific as possible to the demands of hockey. On-ice testing, while less scientific and reliable than laboratory testing, is valid since it measures conditioning in connection with skating technique and mechanical efficiency. Off-ice field tests offer simple, although less sport-specific, ways to assess core strength and flexibility levels. A battery of off-ice laboratory tests provide the most valid and reliable results.

Teams might test at training camp to evaluate the effectiveness of, and a player's commitment to, a summer conditioning program. Midseason retesting is a good way to check if players are maintaining their conditioning levels throughout the season. Retesting during the season can help coaches refine practices and workouts, and determine the recovery needs of players. This information can be especially important at playoff time. Although we no longer test midseason, we do retest players six weeks prior to the playoffs so results can be used to individualize player conditioning and help them "peak" at the right time. Data from postseason testing can indicate what to emphasize when designing the player's off-season conditioning program.

Strength and Flexibility Tests

The following off-ice tests offer ways of assessing the general fitness of players. These simple tests require little equipment and can be done quickly.

Controlled Push-Up Test

Upper-body strength and endurance is important for shooting, bodychecking, warding off opponents, and withstanding full hits. To do the test, the player begins face down in a prone position with the hands on the floor beneath the shoulders. While keeping the body straight and aligned, the arms are straightened until fully extended and then flexed, lowering the body until the nose touches the floor. The player does as many repetitions as possible to complete fatigue, at a rate of 25 per minute (one push-up per 2.4 seconds). A metronome set at 50 clicks per minute will help to maintain a proper pace. The test is discontinued when the athlete cannot fully extend the arms or drops too quickly.

Controlled Sit-Up Test

Core strength assists all on-ice movements and is key to injury prevention. The player lies on the floor with the knees bent to approximately 90 degrees. The feet are flat on the floor (ankles or feet are not held down). Fingertips are placed at the side of the head over the temples. The player sits up and touches elbows to knees and then lowers back down under control, at a rate of 25 repetitions per minute (one per 2.4 seconds). A metronome set at 50 clicks per minute will help to maintain a proper pace. The test is discontinued when the heels lift off the floor, the elbows do not reach the knees, the fingertips slip off the temples, or the player loses the pace to "bounce" up off the floor.

Grip Strength Test

Strength in the hand, wrist, and forearm is important during shooting and puck control. A hand grip dynamometer produces a grip strength measure that correlates well with overall upper-body strength. The dynamometer is held in one hand at the side of the body. The player grips as hard as possible for two or three seconds then relaxes. It is OK if the arm is moved a bit while exerting force. Two efforts are made with each hand and the highest one recorded for each hand.

Sit-and-Reach Flexibility Test

Trunk flexibility reduces the risk of lower back muscle and joint injury. The sit-and-reach test provides an indication of lower back and hamstring flexibility. The player sits without shoes with the legs fully extended. The player slowly bends at the waist and reaches forward with the arms fully extended and palms facing down. To obtain the sit-and-reach measurement, the bottom of the foot is set at the 10-inch (25.4-cm) mark (this is to avoid negative scores when producing normative data). Reaching past the feet results in a score above 10 (25.4), measured with a ruler from the bottom of the feet to the fingertips. If the fingertips do not reach the feet, the score will be less than 10 (25.4). Each player gets three trials. Record the highest score. Players should be warmed up prior to this test.

Anthropometry

The relation of body fat to lean muscle mass is an indicator of general fitness, and is very important for efficient movement and agility on the ice. Body composition is estimated through skinfold assessments. Sub-cutaneous fatfolds are measured by a skinfold caliper.

We use six skinfold sites (biceps, triceps, subscapular, supriliac, anterior thigh, and medial calf) which are summed to represent fat deposits. Various mathematical equations are available to estimate percent body fat, but because of the discrepancy between equation results and the very skinfold sites used, we rely on just the sum as an indication of overall body fat. Skinfold assessments are highly susceptible to tester error, so it is important to make use of an exercise physiologist or other sport scientist who is well versed in the administration of this test.

Hydrostatic weighing is an even more valid and reliable test, producing percent body fat and lean body weight values. We also measure height and weight each time we test athletes.

Fitness Tests for Hockey Conditioning

The following three on-ice tests provide simple ways of determining hockey-specific conditioning. Over the years, hundreds of coaches have asked me for percentile norms that rank results from these tests for players of different ages and levels so they can compare their players to international performance standards. Although I have gathered a great deal of data, additional results are needed to validate my initial rankings. If your test is carefully and successfully administered and you wish to submit the results for inclusion in the calculation of norm tables, I will see that the information is made available for your use once a larger population sample is included. Send your results to Pete Twist, c/o Vancouver Canucks, 800 Griffiths Way, Vancouver, BC, CANADA V6B 6G1. Make sure to include the age and level of players.

Repeat Sprint Skate

The Repeat Sprint Skate (RSS) is an on-ice assessment of anaerobic preparation (anaerobic power and anaerobic endurance), the endurance capabilities of the skating muscles, linear skating speed, recovery ability, and skating efficiency. The test consists of six maximal velocity skating sprints of 91.45 meters repeated every 30 seconds.

To perform the test, the player is positioned behind the red line and starts on the whistle, sprinting to the far red line and coming to a complete stop over the red line. The player immediately reverses direction and sprints to the blue line closest to the starting red line. A timer (A) stands at the far red line and times how long it takes the player to sprint from red line to red line. A second timer (B), at the blue line closest to the starting red line, times the sprint from beginning to end. (see figure 8.1)

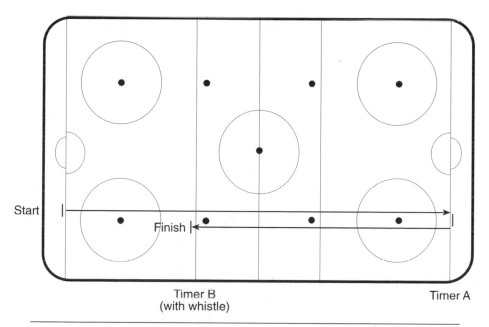

Figure 8.1 Repeat sprint skate

Depending on the time it takes for the player to complete one full sprint interval, whatever remains of the 30-second sprint segment can be used for rest and recovery. For instance, if a player takes 18 seconds to sprint 91.45 meters, he or she gets 12 seconds rest before the next sprint interval begins. The player must be ready at the red line for another sprint interval at the end of the 30 seconds. A 5-second verbal warning is given prior to each repetition. There are three RSS measurements:

1. The *speed index* (usually the first complete length of the ice, from red line to red line) represents anaerobic power performance (ATP-PC system) and full linear speed abilities.

2. The *total time* for the six repetitions represents the player's anaerobic endurance.

3. The *drop-off index*, from the time difference between the slowest and fastest repetitions (usually the first and the last rep), is an indication of anaerobic fitness. If a player's drop-off time is short, the coach knows that the player has come to camp physically prepared. A long drop-off time indicates that the player is in need of improvement. Players should aim to keep their drop-off time within 10 to 15 percent of their speed index. To calculate drop-off index:

$$\text{drop-off index} = \frac{\dfrac{\text{slowest speed}}{\text{repetition time}} - \dfrac{\text{fastest speed}}{\text{repetition time}}}{\text{slowest speed repetition time} \times 100}$$

Here are some helpful tips on administering the test:

- All timers should start their stopwatches on the whistle. One timer (usually B) counts down the last five seconds to ready each player and ready each timer and blows the whistle to start each sprint repetition.

- Players must begin with their feet behind the red line. The speed index sprint is completed when one foot crosses the far red line, but the player must come to a full stop with both feet. The full repetition ends when one foot crosses the blue line at timer B.

- Players usually get 12 to 15 seconds rest between repetitions.

- Once players understand that a drop-off index is being measured, they may pace themselves to manipulate their times for a better drop-off index. To ensure a maximal effort, the speed index should be determined with a one-rep speed test prior to announcing the RSS test. The RSS is administered another day and the speed index is cross-referenced with the speed index measurement from the one-rep speed test. They should be almost identical.

Blue-to-Blue Explosive Start Test

This test measures explosive acceleration using the ATP-PC energy system. To perform the test, the player starts with hips and shoulders in line with the blue line and both feet on the line. One coach stands behind the skater and slaps his stick on the ice to signal the start—eliminating any visual cues for the skater—and the player sprints blue line to blue line. The other coach (or testing assistant) acts as timer and stands even with the far blue line. The timer starts the stopwatch when the starter's stick hits the ice. The time is stopped as the skater's first foot crosses the far blue line. Time is recorded to the nearest 1/10th of a second. The final test result is the average of three attempts. If one of the times differs greatly, it is likely due to tester error. Throw it out and have the skater repeat a fourth sprint after a few minutes rest. The entire team should be taken through their first repetition before the players attempt their second sprint, to provide adequate rest intervals between reps.

The distance from blue line to blue line should be 60 feet. If this differs in your arena, measure out 60 feet and mark the distance with cones, to ensure the standardized test distance.

T-Test

The T-Test is an on-ice assessment of explosive power, the ATP-PC energy system, agility, "quick feet," lateral movement, and acceleration and deceleration ability. These attributes are important in hockey for stop-and-starts, one-on-one confrontations, races for loose pucks, and directional changes.

This test uses two timers per skater and the result will be the average of their times. To prepare for the test, the skater straddles the center red line, facing the timers. The player "self-starts" the test—the timers watch the player's feet and start their watches when one foot begins to move. (see figure 8.2)

The player begins by sprinting to the left to the blue line, either crossing over at the takeoff, or turning and skating forward—whatever style and strategy is preferred. At the blue line, the player must stop completely, facing the timers. For the sprint to be timed complete, one of the player's skates has to cross completely over the blue line (you should position a "line checker" at each blue line to ensure this is done). If one skate does not cross the blue line, the line checker informs the timers, and the test is repeated after a brief rest.

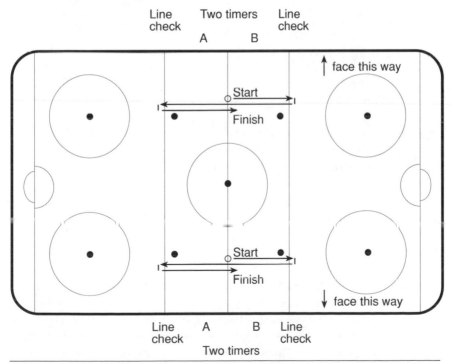

Figure 8.2 T-Test set up with two skaters, four timers, and four line checkers.

The player then skates to the right to the opposite blue line. Again, one foot must cross the blue line and the skater must stop completely, facing the timers. The players then skates left, back to the center red line. The timers stop the test when one foot crosses the center red line.

When measuring the test, both timers start their stopwatches at the same time, and stop their watches as they view the skater cross the finish line. To be as accurate as possible, the timers must concentrate and watch the feet for initiation of movement at the start. Likewise, they have to be ready to stop their watch as the player approaches the finish line. The explosive nature of this test makes it a challenge to measure accurately, and the short distance amplifies the effect of any timing errors. Timers should first practice timing a self-start and a finish.

If the two timers' results are close when measuring the test (for example, 7.04 seconds and 7.10 seconds), the average of the two scores is used. If the two times differ greatly, say by as much as a half second, then there has been tester error. When this happens, and one timer realizes he or she made a mistake, then the other timer's score can be recorded. If the cause of the discrepancy is not clear, have the skater repeat the test after a few minutes rest.

With enough timers and line checkers, two players can be tested at once, one on each side of the ice. Rotate through all the players, then repeat the test, this time starting in the other direction (to the right). Also, as you move through the players, vary their exact starting position across the center red line so the same strip of ice is not continually cut up.

YEAR-ROUND CONDITIONING

As I mentioned in chapter 1, the schedule and design of your year-round conditioning is called *periodization*, which simply means conditioning in cycles where different physical components are developed at different densities, intensities, frequencies, durations, and loads. Periodization is based on scientific principles and methodologies, presenting the best time and the best method for conditioning each physical component.

Periodized conditioning optimizes results, prevents overtraining, and structures your routine so that you peak at selected times. It organizes your on-ice and off-ice practices to prepare you for hockey games. Periodization is both for the long term and the short term. It can involve summer work-outs that key on preparing for a September training camp, but it also includes being ready and rested for each game

Tim Hunter

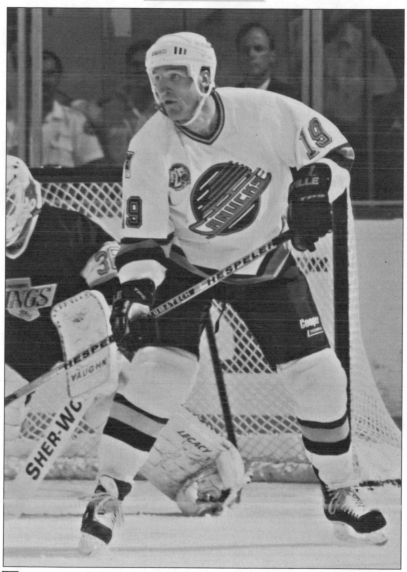

Tim Hunter is the type of player who arrives early and stays late. He works extra hard and always does more than is expected. This provides good leadership for a team, a tremendous role model for young aspiring players, but it also rewards him personally. Hunter has enjoyed 15 years playing the game he loves at the NHL level. He won a Stanley Cup with the Calgary Flames in 1989 and helped Vancouver to the finals in 1994. The same year, at age 34, Hunter was our team's best conditioned player and tied with Kirk McLean for most improved. In 1995, Hunter again received the Top Conditioned Player award.

"There's no question that it's possible to improve, because at my first training camp I was young and slim and in pretty good shape, or what I thought at the time was good condition. I was eager, had a lot of energy, and I saw that players, older players especially, took conditioning very lightly and weren't eager to condition. They didn't think it was very important. I saw that as a way of putting me above everyone else, because with conditioning everyone starts out on a level playing field. We all have the same ability to go out and work hard, be disciplined, and sacrifice to work on our conditioning. Everyone has those potential capabilities to start with, but not everyone is *willing* to do what it takes. I thought if I was willing to commit myself to hard work, spending extra time on the bike, working harder than the next guy, doing more than what was required of me, I'd be in better condition than 90 percent of the guys I was playing against and that would give me the edge. Personally, not having a lot of talent, I thought the conditioning part of the game would give me an edge and help me get my foot in the door. All I've done is build on that every year.

The key to improving is to push yourself both physically and mentally. *Mentally* includes tolerating intense efforts, but it also means not letting confidence or self-esteem or pride limit improvement—it's important for athletes to be willing to try things they are not very good at and to push the limits of things they are already good at. "If you're not making mistakes trying, then you're not trying to improve," says Hunter. "Take the quick-feet drills you do with us on the ice and in the gym. I feel like an imbecile trying to do a sequence of drills I've never done before, moving my feet faster than I ever have before, but once I get doing it, I feel more comfortable. That's a good feeling—to push myself past the comfort zone and improve, and come to know I can improve—that's what it's all about."

The approach to physical preparation has definitely changed during Hunter's pro career, for both teams and individual players. "The *teams* are approaching it as if they have a valuable asset," explains Hunter. "They want to protect their investment in players, field the most competitive team possible, and get injured players back in the game as fast as possible and in the best condition possible. Reconditioned properly, not just back as quick as possible just to get the product back on the ice in any way possible," he adds. "I think in hockey today, you have to rehabilitate your injuries in a hockey atmosphere, not just in a clinic or a doctor's office. Bring your rehabilitation back onto the ice and work on it on the ice. That's what's great, the drills you've showed us on the ice, strengthening drills on the ice or in the gym, specific for that injury to get us back playing in the whole realm of a hockey game as opposed to us just sitting in the clinic or in the medical training room."

"*Players* now see the opportunity in the summer to make themselves better hockey players by training for hockey. Everything is geared towards getting better as a hockey player. Not so much as getting in shape, but getting better as a hockey player. You can become a better hockey player from one season to the next, *in* the summer, by working on things in the off-season geared towards your hockey skills. Stickhandling, specific strength training, quick-hand drills, quick-feet drills . . . everyone's looking for an edge."

of the season. In-season game readiness really tests your periodization skills, because the game schedule; travel; practice intensity, volume, and frequency; practice content; injuries and illnesses; and, in some cases, PR events, media, demotions, call-ups, and trades are all factors that influence when and how a player should be conditioned. Coaches in charge of conditioning may have three hours a day with some players. At other times and with other players, they may only have 10 minutes at the end of practice to work on quickness and agility.

Hockey players are deconditioned throughout a season. The games are intense, and the season is grueling. Hockey demands a lot out of the body for optimal performance. The constant wear and tear on the body results in fatigue that can make in-season maintenance of physical components extra challenging. Players who do not undertake an in-season conditioning program are commonly detrained by playoff time. Hockey, while drawing upon strength and aerobic fitness, does not present the right loads to build them up. Periodizing helps maintain conditioning levels through to the playoffs; it prevents players from losing strength and fitness they have gained over the summer. In this way, periodization also prevents undertraining and helps to maintain in-season conditioning levels. Scheduled carefully, you can even make good gains during the in-season. During the 1993-94 hockey season, Adrien Plavsic of the Canucks gained 14 pounds of lean muscle mass with no increase in body fat, while improving stride power. He accomplished this by following a precise method and timing of conditioning and by being willing to work hard to improve.

Coaching books in all sports break periodization down into different categories. The *macrocycle* is the entire year of conditioning. In some sports it can be longer. For Olympic athletes, the macrocycle would be four years long. The macrocycle is broken down into several distinct phases called *mesocycles*. For hockey, the mesocycles may be the off-season, preseason, in-season, and postseason. These are different periods in which conditioning is structured and organized to build up selected physical attributes while allowing for game schedules and rest and recovery needs. Within each mesocycle are *microcycles*, most of them one week long. Microcycles help you plan a weekly schedule to meet the goals of the mesocycle.

For your needs, to get you headed in the right direction, you need to recognize the different phases or cycles within a year-round hockey conditioning program and to understand that *what* is conditioned and *how* it is conditioned varies in each phase. One phase may concentrate on building the anaerobic energy systems and speed, using specific intensities, exercises, frequencies, volumes, loads, foot contacts, movement patterns, and other variables to manipulate the training effect. Within each phase, for each physical component within a phase, and for each individual athlete, there are specific rules and rates of progression. As you progress from one training cycle to another, the variables are structured to achieve the goals of that specific cycle.

The hockey player's year is divided into four phases. This includes an off-season that may be four to ten weeks long, a preseason of four to six weeks, an in-season that includes exhibition games, regular season games, and playoffs, and a two- to four-week postseason that acts as a transition from the end of the season to when off-season conditioning begins. The exact length and timing of each phase varies with the level of hockey and each team's success level. Players on NHL teams who do not make the playoffs finish their season April 15 and have almost five months until their next training camp. When we went to the seventh game of the Stanley Cup Championship, we were left with only $2^{1}/_{2}$ months between playoffs and training camp, and this included the postseason recovery period! Each team and each player will have to adjust the four phases of conditioning to suit the characteristics of their season.

The physical components targeted in a hockey player's annual conditioning program are shown in figure 8.3. The base of the triangle is the building block, and then various components are progressively

Jeremy Roenick

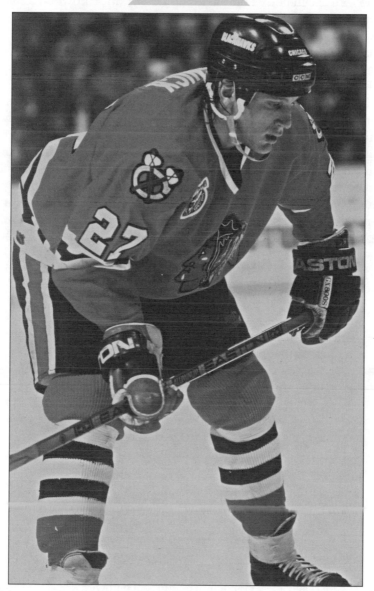

After leading Team USA in scoring and being named to the First All-Star Team at the World Junior Championships, Jeremy Roenick broke into the NHL and was voted the *Sporting News* Rookie of the Year by NHL players. He also competed in the 1991 Canada Cup for Team USA. "For conditioning, I do some upper-body strength work, but I focus more on the lower half of my body. I do a lot of rollerblading and plyometrics in the summer to build my leg strength, endurance, speed, and quickness. Conditioning and quickness drills could be the difference between beating someone to a loose puck or beating someone to the goal on a breakaway. In today's game, speed and quickness are crucial."

Players at all levels can improve, but some players are always trying to learn and constantly trying to improve, while other athletes aren't. "I think it's all in your head," says Roenick. "You have to be willing to do it. You have to have the heart to do it. And you have to have fun while doing it. In order to be an NHL player and be the best you can be, you have to be totally devoted to it, and that means having fun and working hard at it. If you're doing it and think it's a chore, and you're not having fun at it, then you should probably find something else to do."

conditioned, leading to peak hockey performance. The physical demands of hockey are complex and varied, and hockey requires very specific conditioning to transfer to on-ice performance. Factor in

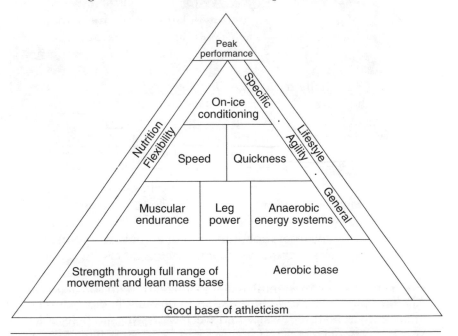

Figure 8.3 Progression from a base of fitness to sport-specific conditioning, building to peak hockey performance.

the different off-seasons, the in-season schedule, and the individual developmental needs of each player, and the coach is presented with an interesting challenge in designing a periodized conditioning program.

OFF-SEASON PREPARATION PHASE

The off-season is spent building a general base of aerobic fitness and a base of strength. Later high-intensity anaerobic conditioning, speed development, muscular endurance and power, and on-ice activity will rely on a solid aerobic and strength base. If the athlete has a short off-season period (five weeks or less), I have them begin working on their aerobic base and strength base at the same time.

Conditioning is structured slightly differently for players with a longer off-season. If your season ends in February or March, as it will for many college teams, or in April, as it will for many other levels, players will have a full postseason, a full six-week preseason, and still be left with a long off-season. Players don't need longer than a six-week preseason, so any leftover time can be added to the off-season phase. For off-season periods of six weeks or more, begin with full strength training and limit aerobic conditioning to twice per week. "When you combine both for extended periods, strength will suffer while the aerobic base will continue to build," says Coach Goldenberg of the Ottawa Senators. Many coaches are concerned that too long a period of aerobic training can slow strength and power growth and detract from high-velocity movements. "I usually try to allow for three to four weeks of strength training without any aerobic work," says Goldenberg. If you have the luxury of a long off-season, first get working on your strength base and lean muscle mass gains, then build strength and aerobic base together over the last five weeks of the off-season. Limiting a heavy schedule of aerobic conditioning to the last five weeks of the off-season addresses the concern that too long a period of continuous aerobic workouts ultimately practices recruiting muscles for slow movements and detracts from high-velocity contraction capabilities. But this is also already accounted for by incorporating intermittent aerobic workouts, which are high-speed, high-intensity workouts that recruit fast-twitch muscle fibers and use high-speed contractions. Initially, expending all of your efforts toward strength training will maximize strength and mass gains. Then, limiting the heavy aerobic period to five weeks and using intermittent aerobic workouts will build the important aerobic base while keeping your body's physical changes more specific to the demands of hockey.

During the off-season, players should stretch daily to complement full range of motion strength training and to improve their flexibility for on-ice speed, quickness, and agility. The off-season is the time to learn and rehearse techniques and movement patterns for quickness, agility, and speed development. These are done at a slow, easy pace as part of warm-ups and cooldowns. This is the time to identify potential strength imbalances and technique flaws that can be worked on in the off-season to enhance future high-intensity drill technique and skill execution.

OFF-SEASON CONDITIONING GUIDELINES

Flexibility
- Stretch daily before and after each workout.

Aerobic
- Complete the aerobic workout no more than twice a week before the last five weeks of the off-season phase.
- Complete the aerobic workout three to five times a week over the last five weeks.
- Begin with continuous aerobic workouts.
- Progress by increasing the duration of each workout. Next, increase the intensity, completing at a faster pace.
- Progress to intermittent aerobic workouts.

Strength
- Complete the strength workout three to four times per week.
- Use moderate weights and high reps (12 to 15) for a one-week break-in period.
- Progress to low reps (6 to 8) and heavy weights.
- As you adapt to the program, increase the volume (number of exercises and number of sets) in the workouts.
- Next, increase the amount of weight you use for each exercise.
- As you increase the intensity of strength workouts, you'll need to decrease volume.
- In the last week of the off-season, begin to decrease the rest intervals between sets.

Anaerobic
- Complete anaerobic sprints once a week as a break-in process.

Quickness and Agility
- Incorporate submaximal quickness and agility movement patterns into warm-ups and cooldowns to give time to assess techniques

and to safely learn movement patterns. This will make future preseason high-intensity work more efficient.

Speed

- This too is sometimes built into the warm-ups and cooldowns, as well as into aerobic runs. Speed is high-quality training, so introduce the techniques involved with various plyometric, overspeed, and resisted-speed exercises at an easy pace. This will allow higher quality speed training in the preseason phase.

Plus

- Other sports that involve constant movement along with directional changes and lateral movement (e.g., soccer, tennis, or basketball) may be used. I recommend staying off the ice throughout the off-season, unless your skating skills are quite poor. If this is the case, on-ice drills, powerskating, and a skating treadmill may be beneficial. Even poor skaters may be better off staying off the ice until the preseason. Practicing skating technique will yield few results without first developing the proper physical attributes needed to support skill execution. Use the off-season time to build the physical tools that can be harnessed to enhance skating technique in the preseason. You need structured conditioning to prepare specifically for hockey, but sometimes you can replace or complement workouts with other sport activities and still get benefits, plus a bit of variety in your program. For example, an intense, well-skilled 70-minute tennis or squash match may replace an aerobic workout and a quickness and agility workout, or complement it by following the tennis or squash match with a shorter 20-minute aerobic workout and a smaller volume of specific quickness and agility drills.

PRESEASON PREPARATION PHASE

Preseason conditioning is characterized by a shift to high-intensity work, explosive movements, high speeds, intervals, and sport-specificity. Figure 8.4 shows the relative change in volume, intensity, technique, and specificity as a player progresses from the off-season through the preseason and into the regular season. As they move into the preseason, players key on the anaerobic energy systems, quickness and agility, and speed, and they continue working on flexibility. Aerobic and strength components are conditioned less frequently, aiming at maintenance while allowing time for more important sprint work. Strength is trained differently, to develop muscular power and muscular endurance, building off of the base of strength and lean muscle mass.

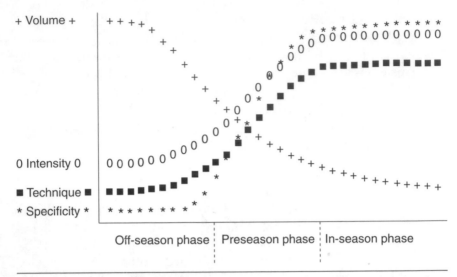

Figure 8.4 The relationship between volume, intensity, technique, and specificity at different times of the season.

PRESEASON CONDITIONING GUIDELINES

Flexibility
- Continue stretching daily.

Aerobic
- Complete the aerobic workout twice a week.
- Consider using continuous workouts as a break from all of the interval training athletes do in this preseason phase. Continuous aerobic workouts also help with recovery from the intense anaerobic workouts.

Strength
- Reduce strength workouts to twice a week.
- Slightly decrease load and increase number of reps to 8 to 15 per set.
- Make exercises more sport-specific, especially in the movement patterns.
- Increase the speed of movement for power.
- Shorten the between-set rest intervals for muscular endurance.

Anaerobic
- Increase anaerobic workout frequency to three times per week.
- Progress by increasing the length of the sprint interval time.
- Next, start to decrease the length of the recovery interval time.
- Next, increase the number of sprint repetitions you're completing.
- In the last portion of the preseason period, do anaerobic sprints on the ice.

Quickness and Agility

- Complete high-intensity quickness and agility workouts twice a week.
- Workouts can be done both off-ice and on-ice throughout the preseason.

Speed

- Speed is conditioned twice per week.
- Start with off-ice sprint drills, resisted speed, overspeed, and plyometrics.
- Sprint drills can be done on-ice during the last half of the preseason phase.

Plus

- Other sports that demand rapid directional and rotational movements can complement your quickness and agility development as well as your anaerobic ATP-PC energy system. High-intensity, high-tempo tennis, squash, racquetball, and badminton are good options. Small group soccer (e.g., four-on-four on a smaller field), two-on-two volleyball, and three-on-three basketball are also suitable.
- Practice on-ice skill work—puckhandling, passing, shooting, skating, angling, etc.
- Scrimmages.

The progression of on-ice activity, from your first on-ice session through readiness to full-intensity scrimmages, is outlined in figure 8.5.

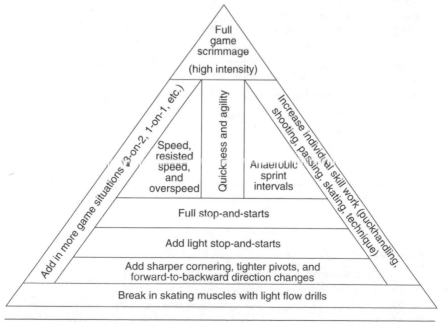

Figure 8.5 Preseason on-ice progression.

IN-SEASON PHASE

The length and complexity (game schedule, travel, tournaments, play-offs) of each team's in-season varies. However, the common theme of in-season conditioning is *maintenance*. Even if the entire summer is spent preparing for hockey, players who do not commit to in-season conditioning are deconditioned by the end of the season. If players don't schedule maintenance workouts, they'll have a lower level of conditioning by playoff time—exactly when optimal conditioning is most important! Some physical components are maintained or improved by the on-ice activity. Other components need to be maintained off the ice—aerobic power and muscular strength are drawn upon for hockey performance, but a hockey game does not provide the specific stimulus needed to build these components.

During the in-season, my goal for athletes is to maintain their overall level of conditioning, plus improve *one* aspect of their game. Considering coaches' evaluations of players and fitness test results, I select one weakness to key on. One player may be given the goal to improve footwork and quickness; another may target improving anaerobic endurance or reducing body fat. Improving one aspect of a player's game may sound simple, but working in the required time in the face of heavy game, practice, and travel schedules, along with fatigue and minor injuries, presents a great challenge for both coach and athlete.

Improving one main area for each player will have a tremendous effect on each athlete's play and the team as a whole. It takes only incremental improvements to make a big difference on team performance. If you improve one thing for each player, and sum these improvements as a team, the result is surprising.

In-season conditioning has different forms and different roles. It may involve conditioning within on-ice practice drills, off-ice conditioning practices, plus extra on-ice and off-ice conditioning on game days for players not in the lineup. It plays a role for injured players, aggressively rehabilitating injuries and bringing the player to full game readiness. Players shouldn't have to "play themselves into shape" in the first few games after returning from an injury. They should return to the lineup in better shape and more game ready than anyone else on the team. Other players have been wearing down their body from games—the injured player has had all that time to build up and improve specific physical and skill areas.

Conditioning also emphasizes rest and recovery. This includes adequate rest intervals between on-ice drills and off-ice conditioning, monitoring the intensities of practices, tracking each player's ice time during games, postgame recovery, and scheduling complete rest days. Workouts may be completed after an evening game specifically to assist in recovery, or to fit in a strength workout so players can take the next day off for rest and recovery. Working toward optimal in-season conditioning does not always mean activity and intense work. Often it may require scheduling light recovery workouts and days of complete rest.

IN-SEASON CONDITIONING GUIDELINES

Flexibility
- Continue flexibility workouts daily, both before and after practices and games.

Aerobic
- Complete off-ice continuous aerobic workouts to maintain aerobic power. These workouts are shorter (20 to 30 minutes) and less frequent (twice a week) but still use high intensity.
- Complete some of the aerobic workouts with a lighter intensity to speed up postgame recovery. These workouts usually last 20 minutes at 70 percent maximum heart rate.

Strength
- Complete short strength workouts twice a week for maintenance.
- During the season, grip strength and leg strength do not suffer great decrements. Some players maintain or build these areas from on-ice activity, while others suffer slight decreases. But all players commonly lose significant upper-body strength over a season. For maintenance purposes, consider spending at least 75 percent of workouts on upper-body strength and abdominal work, and the rest on legs. (You may have players below average in leg strength or stride power who need more time for in-season leg strength).
- Decrease the volume of workouts while keeping the same high intensity. Due to the fatigue or general soreness from physical contact in games, a lot of players feel more comfortable using slightly lighter loads. To accommodate a lighter weight, the between-set rest periods, repetitions per set, and speed of movement can be manipulated to still overload the muscles and stimulate adaptations. You can use lighter loads and faster movements, lifting right up to full fatigue each set—this will help maintain some strength while also building muscular power and muscular endurance. Or, use lighter loads with slow eccentric contractions

("negatives") to help overload the muscle and maintain strength. Lowering rest times between sets is another option that will allow some strength maintenance and muscular endurance benefits while using lighter weights.

- Be flexible. Depending on the game schedule, a strength workout may be a 45-minute workout on a practice day, or a 5-minute push-up routine in the dressing room after a game.

Anaerobic

- Generally, anaerobic conditioning is covered on the ice in regular practice drills or regular practice conditioning drills.
- When players' ice time is limited, or if they are not dressing for games, add anaerobic sprints on the ice after practice or on the bike. Active players who need to lengthen their shift also add in anaerobic sprints. This may help extend their ability to go full-out for 35 seconds to a longer 45-second shift, for example.

Quickness and Agility

- These should be covered in practice. However, I do have players complete supplemental quickness and agility exercises if this area has been identified as needing improvement or if they are not dressing for several games in a row. Even world-class athletes need to improve quickness. Young players are just beginning to develop, and if they have a sufficient strength base, they can improve rapidly in explosiveness. Older players need to key on this area to help maintain their abilities. With specific practices, my athletes over 30 years old still make good improvements in explosiveness.
- Quickness and agility will not suffer deconditioning during the season, but they are also components that can be easily improved throughout a season with two 10-minute practices per week.

Speed

- I only coach an athlete for speed development if this has been identified as a specific weakness and is the most important area the player needs to develop. There are usually two or three players on a team that above all need to improve their overall speed or stride power. For most players, I stress speed capabilities during the preseason, then leave specific speed to the practice drills and game participation.
- Three exceptions may apply to this general in-season speed periodization guideline. One is including extra speedwork for the very slow player who lacks speed more than quickness. Second, I may incorporate overspeed drills for highly skilled players to work on skill execution at faster speeds. Third, for players who are very fast, you can sometimes use repeated resisted speed intervals on

the ice to efficiently train several components at once—for example, leg power, leg strength and endurance, and the anaerobic energy system.

POSTSEASON TRANSITION PHASE

The postseason begins as soon as the playoffs end. This phase has many purposes. One is to recover from the physical demands of the season. By the end of the playoffs, your body is likely craving rest time. Second, the postseason provides a mental break from stress. A third reason for this period is to provide a transition period from the intensity and stress of the playoffs to the generality of the off-season phase.

Some coaches recommend complete rest almost immediately after the last playoff game. Generally, this is not a good idea. In that last game, the physical challenge, mental stress, emotional demands, and hormonal involvement are all at peak output. Following such intensity, the body needs to gear down gradually, not suddenly. Both mind and body are accustomed to functioning at an all-out level—it's unhealthy to abruptly shut everything down completely. The player should continue some very light workouts or participate in other fun sport activities for at least two weeks to taper down toward passive and active rest, recovery, and relaxation.

As you now realize, there is both an art and a science to periodizing each athlete's development. You need to understand the science behind hockey performance—how the body works and how it adapts to different competition and conditioning stressors. But equally important is understanding the art of creating an optimal program for each player. A successful coach must be able to manipulate many conditioning variables involving numerous factors in a way that remains specific to hockey. There is an art to applying the sport science information, and what you condition during each phase, along with how it is conditioned, is a big part of the *art* of exercise prescription.

SAMPLE WORKOUTS

The following sample practices exemplify single days of conditioning designed with specific purposes in mind.

You are encouraged to design your own workouts that reflect the periodization guidelines, the age and abilities of players, their stage of growth and maturation, plus their training experience and fitness levels. These and other factors may cause you to moderate the application of the activities and their prescription.

OFF-SEASON

Small Group Practice

Purpose: To develop a base of strength and lean muscle mass while focusing on legs and back.

Intensity: High, using heavy weights to complete fatigue every set.

Speed of Movement: 1:4; 1 sec positive phase of lift, 4 sec negative phase (cleans are 1:1).

Between-Set Rest Intervals: 2 to 3 min.

Managing Practice: Players work out with a partner for spotting and assistance with forced reps. Pair inexperienced with experienced players for technique assistance, or pair players of equal strength to facilitate competitive motivations. Complete all sets for an exercise before moving to a new exercise. Alternate leg and back exercises.

Warm-Up: 10 min of dynamic flexibility exercises and light load weight training at 1:1 speed of movement.

Off-Ice Exercises (sets/reps):

1. Squats (4 × 6)
2. Calf Raise (3 × 12)
3. Leg Curls (3 × 8)
4. Speedtraxx Hockey Strides (3 × 10)
5. Walking Lunges (2 × 15)
6. Cleans (3 × 6)
7. Pulldowns (3 × 8)
8. Seated Rows (3 × 8)
9. Good Mornings (2 × 15)

Full Team Practice

Purpose: To provide concurrent conditioning for continuous aerobic, intermittent aerobic, and anaerobic abilities while improving athleticism, single-leg balance, agility, and eccentric decelerating.

Intensity: Moderate.

Speed of Movement: Moderate for hike, faster for flag football intervals.

Between-Set Rest Intervals: 2 min.

Managing Practice: Begin practice with a 45 min hike. Instruct players to alternate between a powerful pushoff up inclines and using hip flexors and hamstrings for stride recovery. Key players in on foot placement and knee/back position for safety and performance, especially on the descent. After the hike, move right into the flag football intervals, emphasizing good effort then rest and recovery. Split your team in half. For a 20-person roster, make two teams of 10. Five from each team play while 5 rest. For 5-on-5 flag football, mark off a small boundary so players rely on agility versus straight linear runs.

Off-Ice Activities:

1. Mountain hiking (45 min)
2. Flag football on small field (2 min on, 2 min rest)
3. Static stretching (each player leads one stretch, for a total of 20 stretches)

Individual Practice

Purpose: To develop leg strength, power, plus provide an anaerobic break-in.

Intensity: High.

Speed of Movement: 1:2 for strength exercises, and full speed for anaerobic sprints.

Between-Set Rest Intervals: 2 min.

Warm-Up: 10 min aerobic bike or stairclimber, plus one light set of squats.

Off-Ice Exercises (sets/reps):

1. Squats (4 × 8)
2. Sumo Side Lunge (1 × 12)
3. Lateral Crossover Box Step Ups (2 × 10)
4. Leg Curls (2 × 10)
5. Speedtraxx Lateral Strides (3 × 12)
6. Speedtraxx Crossover Strides (2 × 10)

Anaerobic Activities:

1. Stair Sprints, 2 steps up, single steps down, continuous up and down to total 30 sec (3 × 30 sec, 1:4 work-to-rest)
2. Stride Length Running Sprints (3 × 30 sec; 1:4 work-to-rest)

PRESEASON

Small Group Practice

Purpose: To develop explosive power, muscular endurance, lactic acid toleration, and maintain strength while focusing on all major muscle groups and explosive movements.

Intensity: High, using light to moderate weights but high-speed efforts.

Speed of Movement: Fast.

Between-Set Rest Intervals: No rest between sets. 1:2 work-to-rest ratio between circuits.

Managing Practice: Players work out in groups of three. One player completes 1 set of each exercise without stopping, then rests while the other players go through the circuit. Each player goes through the circuit 4 times.

Warm-Up: 5 min of aerobic activity, 5 min of dynamic flexibility, 1 light set of cleans and squats, plus individualized static stretching.

Off-Ice Exercises (sets/reps):

1. Powercleans (4 × 10)
2. Medicine Ball Push-Ups (4 × 10)
3. Squats (4 × 15)
4. Abdominal Crunches (4 × 15)
5. Push Press (4 × 10)
6. Hockey Lunges (4 × 15)
7. Weight Plate Stickhandling (4 × 15)
8. Upright Rows (4 × 10)
9. Reverse Curls (4 × 10)
10. Squat Jumps (4 × 15)

Full Team Practice

Purpose: To develop quickness, agility, and speed.

Intensity: High.

Speed of Movement: Explosive.

Between-Set Rest Intervals: 2 min.

Managing Practice: Players are paired up so they can work in partners on shadowing, matching, and resistance drills. Pair up so there is some height difference within each pair. Run one drill at a time. All players are on same drill.

Warm-Up: 10 min dynamic warm-up.

Off-Ice Exercises (sets/reps):

1. Stride Length Match Running (3 × 40 meters)
2. Stride Frequency Match Running (3 × 40 meters)
3. Lateral Bounding (2 × 20 foot contacts)
4. Resisted Linear Sprints (2 × 40 meters)
5. Resisted Angle Sprints (2 × 40 meters)
6. Ankle Tubing Shadowing Drill (4 × 15 sec)
7. React and Sprint Tennis Ball Drops (partner drops ball) With Sideways Start (3 × left; 3 × right)
8. Lateral Line Drills (2 × 10 sec each leg)

Static Stretching Exercises:

1. Kneeling Lower Body Stretch (1 × 40 sec)
2. Seated Groin Stretch (2 × 45 sec)
3. Kneeling Leg Stretch (2 × 30 sec)
4. Standing Calf Stretch (3 × 30 foot contacts)

On-Ice Drills:

1. 5 min dynamic flexibility exercises
2. Partner Flow Puck Race (2 times)
3. Quick Pivot, High Drive to Net (3 times for each side)
4. Forward/Backward Single Transition (10 sec clockwise, rest; repeat counterclockwise)
5. Forward/Backward Lateral Crossover Drill (2 times each way)
6. Lateral Line Drill (2 × 10 sec)
7. Agility Strap Shadowing Drill (4 turns; 2 on offense, 2 on defense)

Individual Practice

Purpose: To develop speed.

Intensity: High.

Speed of Movement: Fast, full-out, explosive movements.

Between-Set Rest Intervals: Individualize; rest until comfortable.

Warm-Up: Half-Speed Sprint Runs (4 × 100 meters) and 5 min dynamic flexibility exercises.

Off-Ice Speed Drills:

1. Lateral Bounding (2 × 20 foot contacts)
2. Lunge Jumps (2 × 20 foot contacts)
3. 5 min dynamic flexibility exercises
4. Full-Speed Runs (2 × 15 sec)
5. Downhill Overspeed Sprints (6 × 10 sec)
6. Overspeed Tubing Sprints (4 × 5 sec)
7. Overspeed Tubing, Sideways Start (6 × 5 sec; 4 times off weaker side, 2 times off superior side. For instance, 4 sprints starting to the left, and 2 sprints starting to the right)
8. 10 min static stretching exercises

On-Ice Speed Drills:

1. 5 min dynamic flexibility exercises
2. Flow Speed Drill (start 2 times from left corner, 2 times from right)
3. Speed Change-Up Drill (2 × 20 sec)
4. 5 min static stretching exercises
5. Full-Speed Sprints With Skating Start (2 times)
6. Let-Goes (3 times)
7. Overspeed Tubing Forward (3 times)
8. Overspeed Tubing, Sideways Start (4 times off weaker side, 2 times off stronger side)
9. 5 min dynamic flexibility exercises
10. 10 min static stretching exercises

IN-SEASON

Small Group Practice

Purpose: To provide additional conditioning and quickness/agility development for players who have not been receiving a lot of game time recently (zero to 12 min per game). Focus on quality, technique, and overspeed during the on-ice quickness and agility practice. Emphasize full efforts, fighting through fatigue, and lactic acid toleration during the anaerobic bike sprint intervals.

Intensity: High.

Speed of Movement: Fast.

Managing Practice: On-ice, six players complete a drill one at a time, for a 1:5 work-to-rest ratio. Give 90 sec between tag drills. Complete the quickness and agility drills before the team practice, while players are fresh. Complete the bike sprints after the team practice.

Warm-Up: 10 min of light aerobic activity and 5 min of light on-ice activity.

On-Ice Quickness and Agility Drills:

1. Two-Step Forward/Backward Circles (2 sets left, 2 sets right; twice around circle each set)
2. Quick Pivot, Low Drive to Net (3 times each side of ice)
3. Quick-Feet Coach Directions (2 times)
4. Tag: very small boundary (6 times, once with each player starting)

Regular Full Team Practice

Anaerobic Bike Sprints:

1. Bike aerobic pace for 5 min.
2. Sprint full speed, heavy resistance, for 45 sec.
3. Bike light aerobic pace, light resistance, for 45 sec recovery.
4. Complete a total of 6 sprints and relief intervals, all at 1:1 work-to-relief ratio.
5. Bike aerobic pace for 10 min recovery.

Static Stretching:

1. Lying Knee to Chest Stretch (2 × 30 sec)
2. Lying Gluteal Stretch (1 × 30 sec)
3. Seated Hamstring Stretch (2 × 45 sec)
4. Standing Quadricep/Hip Flexor Stretch (1 × 30 sec)

Full Team Postgame Practice

Purpose: To provide overall strength maintenance, and develop muscle endurance and quick feet.

Intensity: High.

Speed of Movement: 1:1 for strength exercises, explosive for quickness drills.

Between-Set Rest Intervals: No rest between stations.

Managing Practice: Players begin this circuit as soon as they are ready after the game. If you get several players ready to go at once, start a couple of players at station #7 and also #12, two abdominal stations, to spread players out and keep them moving through. Other players begin at station #1. They will need a partner for station #2, then can proceed individually. Use moderate loads for all exercises but squat jumps and lateral raises, which use a light load (abdominal exercises and quickness drills use no loading). Go through circuit once. Pick up a partner for #19, then move off to individualized stretching for postgame and postworkout recovery.

Off-Ice Exercises (sets/reps):
1. Full Bent-Leg Sit-Ups (1 × 25)
2. Medicine Ball Chest Pass (1 × 20)
3. Incline Leg Press (1 × 20)
4. Bench Press (1 × 15)
5. Leg Curls (1 × 15)
6. Push Press (1 × 12)
7. Lower Ab Push Press (1 × 25)
8. Pulldowns (1 × 12)
9. Squats Up to Toes (1 × 10)
10. Seated Rows (1 × 12)
11. Squat Jumps (1 × 15)
12. Crunches (1 × 25)
13. Hammer Curls (1 × 12)
14. Two-Foot Lateral Cone Hops (1 × 20 foot contacts)
15. Dips (1 × 15)
16. Lateral Angled Box Jumps (1 × 20 foot contacts)
17. Lateral Raise (1 × 15)
18. Two-Foot Angled Hops (1 × 20 foot contacts)
19. Medicine Ball Chest Pass, Short Distance (1 × 20)
20. 10 min static stretching exercises

Individual Practice

Purpose: To improve aerobic base and decrease body fat while improving athleticism, quick hands, and abdominals and back strength.

Intensity: Moderate.

Speed of Movement: Moderate for aerobic and strength exercises, explosive for quick hand drills.

Between-Set Rest Intervals: 1 min.

Managing Practice: Do these activities following a regular full team practice.

Aerobic Activity: 45 min continuous aerobic bike or stairclimb.

Off-Ice Exercises (sets/reps):

1. Tennis Ball Drops (Overhand catch) (2 × 10 drops)
2. Tennis Ball Drops (Overhand catch to opposite side) (2 × 10)
3. Medicine Ball Shoulder-to-Shoulder Pass (2 sets each shoulder × 20 passes)
4. Medicine Ball Back-to-Back Pass (1 × 25 left, 1 × 25 right)
5. Full Bent-Leg Sit-Ups (2 × 20)
6. Lower Ab Push Press (3 × 15)
7. Trunk Rolls (1 × 60 sec)
8. Speedtraxx Hockey Strides (No hand or chest support) (1 × 20 left, 1 × 20 right)

ABOUT THE AUTHOR

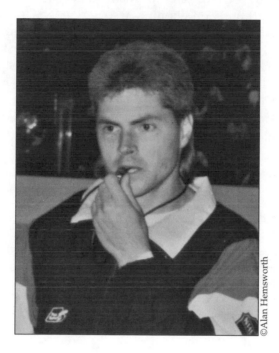

©Alan Hemsworth

Peter W. Twist, one of the foremost conditioning experts in North America, has coached hundreds of hockey players at all levels—from high school to the professional ranks. Twist is strength and conditioning coach for the Vancouver Canucks of the National Hockey League. He also has instructed hundreds of national, international, and professional athletes in a variety of other sports, including football, soccer, tennis, and basketball.

Twist, who earned his MPE degree in coaching science from the University of British Columbia, is president of the Professional and Collegiate Hockey Conditioning Coaches Association. He has lectured extensively on conditioning topics at academic conferences, hockey seminars, and sports banquets.

Coauthor of *The Physiology of Ice Hockey—A Testing and Training Manual*, Twist has helped train such world-class athletes as NHL stars Trevor Linden and Pavel Bure and NBA great Hakeem Olajuwon. Twist also has helped numerous over-30 athletes to become quicker and more agile and to extend their careers. A passionate teacher, Twist lectures to university undergraduate and graduate classes, academic conference audiences, and sport-camp participants. He is the author of numerous articles on player development and conditioning and coeditor of the *Journal of Hockey Conditioning and Player Development*.

Twist is also regional director for the British Columbia branch of the National Strength and Conditioning Association (NSCA) and a member of the National Institute of Speed, Agility and Quickness.

As a varsity hockey player Twist was winner of the Best Defenseman Award at the University of British Columbia and McMaster University. In his leisure time, he enjoys swimming, cycling, and mountain hiking with his wife, Julie, and their dog, Rico.

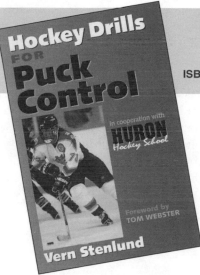
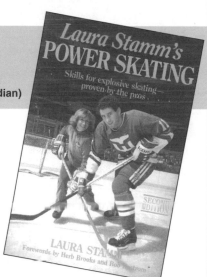